Dr. Poo:
The Scoop on Comfortable Poop

William Sears, MD
and Martha Sears, RN

DR. POO: THE SCOOP ON COMFORTABLE POOP
William Sears, MD and Martha Sears, RN

This book is written as a source of information only. The information contained in this book should not be considered a substitute for the advice of a qualified physician or medical professional. Please consult your healthcare provider before beginning any new healthcare program.

Copyright ® 2018 Regular Girl and Tomorrow's Nutrition. All Rights Reserved. No part of this publication may be reproduced, stored in a retrieval system, or transmitted, in any form or in any means – by electronic, mechanical, photocopying, recording or otherwise – without prior written permission by the copyright holder.

Published by: Regular Girl® and Tomorrow's Nutrition®
Minneapolis, Minnesota
www.RegularGirl.com
www.TomorrowsNutrition.com

ISBN: 978-0-692-05925-8

Printed in Canada

Consult Your Healthcare Provider

Readers, the pooping pointers you read are based on scientific studies and years of medical experience. Yet, you may have special health issues that require a personalized pooping program. Be sure to consult your healthcare provider before doing the suggestions in this book.

DrPoo.com

For more poo learning, join our network of poo stories and updated information about how to poo that is right for you. Join our Perfect Poo Club at DrPoo.com.

Learn More

For a second helping of comfortable pooing information, and supporting scientific references, see AskDrSears.com/DrPoo.

TABLE OF CONTENTS

FOREWORD: BRYCE WYLDE   4

OUR BABY'S STORY   9

MEET DR. POO   12

CHAPTER 1: WHAT'S IN POO? HOW TO POO BETTER   13

A Poo Trip from Top to Bottom * Meet Your Microbiome * *What is Poop Made Of?* * Portrait of a Perfect Poop

CHAPTER 2: THE THREE-STEP PERFECT POOP PLAN FOR BEGINNER POOPERS: INFANTS AND TODDLERS   30

Step 1: Feed Baby the Perfect Milk for Perfect Poo * Step 2: Begin Baby on Poo-Friendly Solids * Poo-Friendly Food Preparation * Step 3: Nibble Your Way to Perfect Poo * *Be Regular!* * Dr. Bill and Martha's Remedy for Baby Constipation

CHAPTER 3: THE FOUR-STEP PERFECT POOP PLAN –FOR ALL AGES   41

Step 1: Chew-Chew Times Two * Step 2: Eat Poo-Friendly Foods * *Best Foods for Better Bowels* * Step 3: Stoolade: Shake it Out – The Top Tip for Pooping Problems * Step 4: Don't Worry, Just Poo! Stress-less Pooping

CHAPTER 4: CURING CONSTIPATION   49

My Pellet-Poop Story * *Dr. Poo's Six-Step Colon Fitness Plan* * Why Chronic Constipation is Dangerous * Dr. Poo's Five-Step Constipation Cure * *Dr. Poo's Recommended Daily Fiber – For All Ages* * In Search of the Perfect Fiber Supplement

CHAPTER 5: ASK DR. POO: MORE QUESTIONS YOU MAY HAVE   59

Poo at School * Holding Poo * Fear of Flushing * Best Pooping Position * Dangle Pooping * Tell-Tale Underwear * Blood Streaks in Poo * Stinky Poo * Tween Poo * Pooping While Pregnant * Green Poo * Gassy Poo * Morning Poo * Pre-Op Poo * Natural Laxatives * *Enjoy a Fiber-Fluid Balance* * Pooping While Traveling * FODMAPs * *Poo Rules – A Summary* * Dr. Poo's Chart

FOREWORD

Early on in my clinical practice, some of the most daunting cases I had were infants and children with constipation, diarrhea and digestion issues. In the last few decades, a more natural approach to these issues has become the popular approach by parents as a first line therapy before considering any over the counter stool loosening agents, suppositories, or drugs offered up by conventional medicine. But, alas, which were proven safe, pure, and effective? I certainly wasn't about to "practice" on these youngest and most vulnerable of my patients.

Luckily, after doing a lot of research, I came across Dr. Bill Sears' series of books in the "Sears Parenting Library". Finally, a doctor who spoke my language and had the experience of successfully treating many thousands of infants and children using natural and—when necessary—conventional medical intervention. This combination approach is known as simply *best* medicine. Most importantly of all, he spoke the language understood by the parents who trusted me with the care of their children. Many hundreds of consultations to follow became: "try this supplement, this nutritional modification, this probiotic, and *definitely* read these books by Dr. Bill Sears." Dr. Bill's teachings became game changers for my personal practice and the lives of my littlest patients and their families.

Twelve years ago, my own life changed forever. I became a father. I have two beautiful young children of my own whom my wife and I have raised to be super healthy using the very principles laid out by Dr. Bill and Martha Sears. I'm writing this foreword and praise, for one very simple reason: I want this for you and your precious children too!

We know that what goes up, must come down. But equally as true and even more important is: what goes in, must come out!

The "must come out" part has been a human fascination since the dawn of man. It has also been a topic many consider taboo. But the process is a very natural part of life and one that has many implications for optimal health.

From your mouth to the toilet bowl and everything in between is very misunderstood and often plain ignored. We are fed by the food industry, which pays little attention to our health. When our digestive system fails, we are treated by the health industry, which pays no attention to food. There is something seriously missing here.

Dr. Poo is here to change all this!

Together, Dr. Bill Sears, M.D., and his wife Martha Sears, R.N., have made it their recent calling to collaborate once again - this time bringing attention to the importance of poo to help bridge the gap between nutrition and health.

Your family doctor or Pediatrician may have asked you about whether your child is "regular", but do you really know what that means? Have you ever questioned the quality, color, or consistency?

What about the experience your child has during a bowel movement? What does it all mean?

Among the many epiphanies you'll have reading this masterful book, you will become intimately familiar with what exactly is in poo (far more than you ever thought!), how to poo better, perfect poo plans for beginner poopers and all ages, as well as learn how to naturally cure constipation for good.

The idea that food is a cornerstone to optimal health is nearly as old as recorded history. You have likely heard Hippocrates' famous quote: "let food be thy medicine and let medicine thy food".

These views have gained many adherents in the last century. What you'll learn in these pages is that besides the popular phrase "you are what you eat," *you are what you poo*! Poo quality is a direct reflection of how healthy you and your loved ones are.

Sadly, to this very day across North America the pharmaceutical industry maintains its control and many conventionally trained doctors remain dismissive of natural and nutritional therapies and interventions. Are doctors ready to think outside the pillbox? Dr. Poo is!

With all the evidence mounting about good and bad bacteria in the gut, the gut-brain connection, and the microbiome and immune health - paradoxically there still remains a significant nutrition gap in North America.

A big issue is that there is a serious disconnect between how patients and doctors perceive diet and its relationship to poo.

There is also a lot of confusion within the realm of nutrition and natural intervention and prevention. From fad diets to unsubstantiated supplements there are so many "nutritional therapies" out there, so many programs with so many claims, and so little science to back them up that it's no wonder that it's hard for sound nutritional therapies to break through.

That is...until now.

Dr. Bill Sears is the foremost expert in pediatric care, health, and nutrition, having helped busy parents raise healthier families for over 40 years. He has authored more than 30 highly acclaimed best-selling books and has decades of experience in clinical practice born out of residencies at two world renowned Children's Hospitals: Boston and Toronto's Sick Children - my own hometown. His incredible wife and collaborator, Martha Sears is no ordinary Registered Nurse. She is also a former childbirth educator, a La Leche League leader, and a lactation consultant. Martha is the co-author of their 25 parenting books and is a popular lecturer and media guest drawing on her eighteen years of breastfeeding experience. If you were a fly on the wall at the Sears' residence (or as lucky as I've been to join them for some exquisite homecooked dinners), you may come to know Martha as "the fixer". They have a lot of incredible ideas, but over their many years together Martha has perfected the art of turning those genius ideas into manageable, grounded, and useful applications that will make you healthier. I would be fully remiss if I didn't mention the experience that comes with raising their eight (yep – 8!) wonderful children together. It is that kind of experience that speaks all on its own!

This latest work, **Dr. Poo: The Scoop on Comfortable Poop**, is the most relevant, useful and comprehensive compilation of the importance of poo you will ever read. In these pages you will find all of Dr Bill's and Martha's best research, personal, and clinical experience complete with innovative programs and techniques to naturally address – and in many cases prevent – digestive issues altogether.

Dr. Poo is incisive and illuminating. We all poop, which means there is something for everyone in this book. So what are you waiting for? Pull up a stool, and start reading. All poo jokes aside (they can get very corny), turn the page, because amongst them awaits the best bowel movement of your life!

- Bryce Wylde
Author of *Wylde on Health*

OUR BABY'S STORY

I'm including this family's story about their young daughter's digestive issues because I know it's relatable to many others. Please keep in mind that every child and condition is unique. What worked for this child may not work for your child. Please consult with your child's healthcare provider. - Dr. Sears

Our beautiful baby girl was born on July 12, 2016. Since birth, she has been a healthy baby, growing and thriving physically, and meeting all her early milestones for cognitive and physical development.

She was about three weeks old when we noticed that she had extreme gas. My husband and I, as first-time parents, relied heavily on doctors for advice and guidance. We tried everything: exercises, bath treatments, Mylicon drops, Gripe water and others. We met with lactation consultants, we tried enzyme drops, probiotics and would even give her milk from a syringe. The gas continued for months.

At seven months, the symptoms of gas began to dissipate and a new problem emerged: she was unable to pass a bowel movement on her own and could not digest solids in any way, shape or form. We felt helpless and no one had any answers. Aside from turning to prayer, and our faith that God would get us through this, we were feeling the pressure of being lost in this situation.

At this point I turned to books. The first book I ordered was a large green tome from Dr. Bill Sears and his family entitled, "The Baby Book."

I immediately felt as if I had someone in my corner. I did more research on Dr. Bill and realized he was down the street from our house! I couldn't believe it! I called and set up an appointment.

Immediately, Dr. Bill explained that he had a way to assist her in regaining her healthy intestinal function. He handed us his new manuscript that was soon to be published, entitled, "Dr. Poo." He introduced me to the microbiome and the connection to fiber, and said that with the correct regimen of probiotics and prebiotics, fiber supplements and diet, she would be going to the bathroom on her own, without severe gas pain, in no time.

My husband and I rushed home to read the Dr. Poo book and get started on the regimen right away. We used the information to create Dr. Bill's recommended smoothie, made with Sunfiber.

About three weeks later, two days before her 14-month birthday, her symptoms started to improve! She started passing gas on her own. She even did what was in accordance with the Dr. Poo book: a healthy poo!

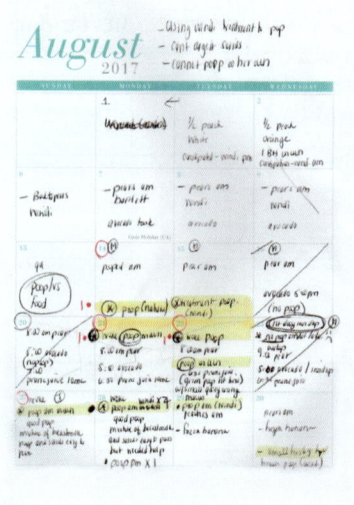 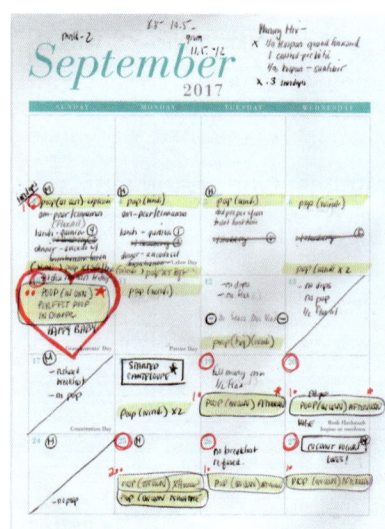

We are blessed and we are a happy family. I can proudly say she is pooing like a champ. For months straight she has been having a healthy poo every day, sometimes two times a day, with a day off here and there. We absolutely LOVE Sunfiber! God Bless Dr. Bill for never giving up and for helping others like us who really need it.

Sincerely,
Grateful parents

MEET DR. POO

When I began pediatric practice in 1972, studying poo was not high on my learning list. Then reality hit. Many of the concerns parents had were about poo: the color, consistency, frequency, shape, and so on. My early years as a doctor and parent were like an on-the-job poo school. I learned that one of my goals as a good doctor was to teach parents how to get their child off to the right poo. In addition, a personal colon-health crisis prompted me to develop a fondness for healthy bowel function.

In addition to witnessing pooping patterns in my 50 years of medical practice, along came eight little Sears poopers and ten grandpoopers. Martha and I estimate we have changed over 5,000 poopy diapers with the full range of poo quality and quantity.

Meet my imaginary partner in pediatric practice, Dr. Poo. During my 50 years as a doctor, I have spent the most time discussing gut concerns – what goes into the top end (food), and what comes out the bottom end (poo). As you learn an important poo point, Dr. Poo will give you the "bottom line" to help you remember it. For example:

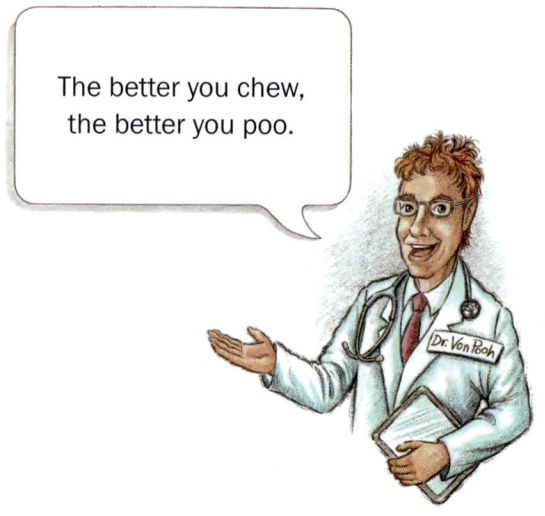

CHAPTER 1
WHAT'S IN POOP? HOW TO POO BETTER

When you poo better you feel better. That's what you want your family to learn. Over my years as a father, grandfather, doctor, and now a self-taught poopologist, I have come to realize that healthy pooing, as we'll nicely call it, is one of the least understood vital signs of having a healthy body. I invite all parents, teachers, and all who care about children's gut health to come with me on a top-to-bottom tour of why we poo, and how to poo more comfortably.

It's a subject we want to hide – literally behind closed bathroom doors. Yet, after reading this book – and following our pooing strategies – you will learn to appreciate what perfect pooing does for your health. As a poo-perk, just by reading – and doing – this book's tips, you will get frequent belly laughs that will literally move things along.

Poo happens. Everyone poos. Poop, for better or worse, is the main cause of your gut feelings – some good, some not so good. When your poop is right, you feel good in your gut; when it's wrong, you don't. Sometimes poop comes out too fast, a messy nuisance called diarrhea; sometimes it gets too hard and stays in too long – a pain in the gut called constipation. By doing the tips in this book, you will have poops to be proud of.

A NOTE FROM DR. BILL: MY PERSONAL POOP STORY

Like many healthcare providers, poop was not near the top of my list of educational objectives. Poop happens! Sometimes too much, sometimes too little, but it is not something most people want to talk or read about. I never realized how medically important it is to have "just the right poo for you" until:

Colon cancer caused me to care. Twenty years ago one big poop change – drops of bright red blood – changed my attitude about poop and why I had to learn more about it as a doctor. And, even more importantly, how to make poopology KISMIF – keep it simple, make it fun. That change of mindset about what's going on down there led to the writing of this book.

Also, now in my 50th year as a doctor, I realized that questions about baby and child poop was near the top of the list of parent concerns. Yet, even as a doctor, I often had no satisfactory answers for parents' questions. Now when a parent asks me about anything to do with their precious child's bowel movements, I eagerly and scientifically can answer their questions.

Poo better, feel better. What really got me excited about one of the very subjects that doctors often avoid happened within a few months of changing my diet – and my attitude about poop. I noticed interesting changes in my poop, and I noticed my good gut feelings before and after my increasingly regular trips to the toilet.

What goes in, must come out. What's in poop is frequently on the no-no list to talk about, especially with younger children – just the opposite of what you will learn in this book. If poop doesn't happen, you would spend each day with a giant pain in the gut. Admittedly, "So, how is your poop…" is probably never going to become a favorite topic of dinner conversation. Yet, after you read this book you will not only be able to poo easier and healthier, you will naturally feel good about one of your body's most important daily "productions."

POOP MATH

Your authors are highly experienced kid-poop observers. Moving onto poop math for adults: Since ideally the average person should poo as frequently as they eat, at least three meals and three poops a day, that translates into an average of a thousand poops a year. And, if you're lucky enough to experience life into old-age, you may pass 100,000 poops in your lifetime. So, since you're going to do it – a lot – you might as well enjoy the healthy version of it. And that's what this book is all about.

A POO TRIP FROM TOP TO BOTTOM

In order to make your poop better so you can feel better, you need to first understand how it's made. Let's follow a meal from the top end of your intestinal tract – your mouth – to when it comes out the bottom end. The top poo lesson for you to learn:

The healthier the food that goes in your top end, the better the poop that comes out the bottom end. Plus, as you will learn, there are tips for improving your total poop experience.

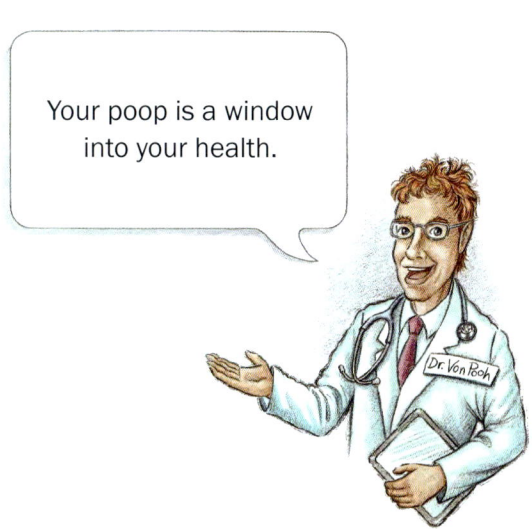

Your poop is a window into your health.

WHAT TO CALL IT

The number of names for poop is rivaled by the number of names for pee. "Poo" and "poop" have survived as the top terms that everyone, including kids, feel less embarrassed talking about. Like "mama" and "dada," it's a word that even young toddlers can say– "poopie."

You are what you eat—you are what you poo. We want to show that there is a cause-and-effect relationship between what and how you eat and what and how you poo.

The better you chew, the better you poo. Good Gut Feelings 101 states that the more predigestion you have occurring in your mouth, the smoother the elimination will be on the bottom end. This begins with one of the first poo lessons I teach my little patients in my pediatric practice: chew-chew times two.

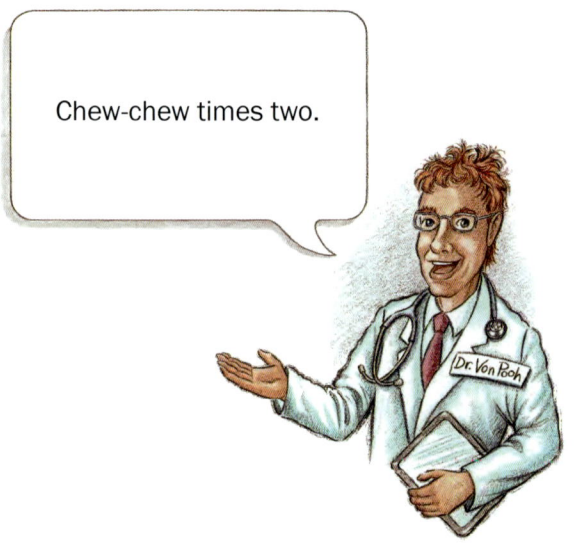

Food must first become "goop" before it forms poop. You take a bite of salad. Because it's full of stringy fiber you need to chew this a lot. The more you chew, the more saliva you make. Meanwhile, down below, your stomach is waiting, and, if your stomach could talk it would say, "Hey mouth, chew a lot and chew slowly because that makes my job easier down here." The chewed salad, which you can now label "goop" (a mixture of the chewed salad and slimy saliva), will eventually become poop. Like wiggly kids on a slip-and-slide, the gooey bite slides down the slippery esophagus into the stomach.

Your body's blender. Your stomach functions as your body's blender, churning and grinding the food until the stomach decides, with the help of messages from other parts of the gut, that the goop is ready to move to the next stop – your small intestines.

Ever wonder why soon after you eat you get the urge to poo? As a tribute to the great design for digestion, there is a nerve pathway going from the stomach to the colon called the "gastro-colic reflex." Imagine that when your stomach gets full, it sends a neurochemical message to the colon saying, "Prepare to evacuate—there is a whole new meal coming down," and the colon obliges.

The small intestine is the largest part of your intestinal tract, so that's where the food being digested spends most of its time. This is necessary because the small intestine is where most of the nutrients from the food are absorbed into the bloodstream to be used for growth, energy, and repair. The lining of the small intestine is like a conveyor belt: as the food passes along, the smart cells lining the intestine are saying to one another, "We need that carb…we need that fat…we need that protein…we need that vitamin," and so on, and one by one they open doors to grab the nutrient they need. They take it in, and further disassemble it into smaller particles and molecules, and then deliver it into the vast vascular highway surrounding the gut to deposit the needed nutrients throughout the body.

As the food being processed travels downward, the gallbladder squirts digestive juices that help break down the stomach-blended food into smaller particles for digestion. The gallbladder supplies a green fluid called bile (an emulsifier) to dissolve fats. Because of this green bile, goop actually starts out green in the small intestine and, as the bile is recycled, the goop turns brown by the time it reaches the large intestine. (Because babies have a faster "transit time"—the time it takes for goop to become poop—an occasional "green poop" is normal.)

Where poop is made. After the small intestine has extracted everything it needs from the digested salad, what's leftover travels onto where poop is made—the large intestine. When it reaches the large intestine, imagine the lower part of your gut dealing with the fibrous part of the salad that the small intestine didn't digest. In fact, the large intestine would say, "We live on your leftovers. Down here we digest what you couldn't up there." And it's the process of recycling this waste that creates poop.

YOU-POO

While it's obvious that no one will share how his pooing is doing on a "You-Poo" channel, everyone's poop is as unique as their personality and diet. Once you've tried our perfect poop program (PPP), you'll continue to feel such good gut feelings that you'll be motivated to continue it. At this writing, I am now eighteen years into my "perfect pooing" lifestyle—and loving it!

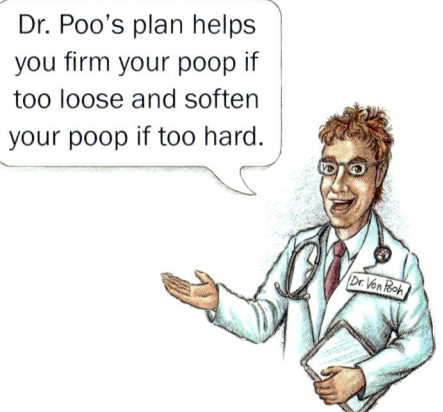

Dr. Poo's plan helps you firm your poop if too loose and soften your poop if too hard.

The final few feet – *the anatomy of evacuation*. When poop arrives at the rectum, which is richly supplied with smooth muscle and nerves, the rectum senses the presence of material that needs to be passed through and evacuated. Two donut-like muscles called *sphincters* work together to push the poop out. The internal sphincter automatically relaxes as if saying to the muscular guard gate: "Relax, man, and let me through."

A second guard gate—the external donut muscle, the one you observe when you give your child a suppository or use a rectal thermometer—has different nerves. This outer muscle, called the external sphincter, is under your control. When you feel the urge to go, this muscle helps prevent embarrassing accidents. You can tell your external donut muscle: "Hold on for a few more minutes until I can get to the bathroom."

These two muscles (the "I got to go" and the "you can hold it") work in harmony with one another. Both have marching orders that say, "Don't stretch us because that weakens us." The donut muscles don't like to be stretched too much for too long (constipation) or they weaken. If this happens, the internal one can't push things along very well and/or the outer one doesn't hold on, so you either retain or leak.

"Colon fitness" is important for two reasons: 1) it's where the most poop is made, and 2) the colon is where exciting new research reveals a new "organ" exists, called your microbiome. (See related sections: Constipation, page 49; and Colon Fitness, page 51).

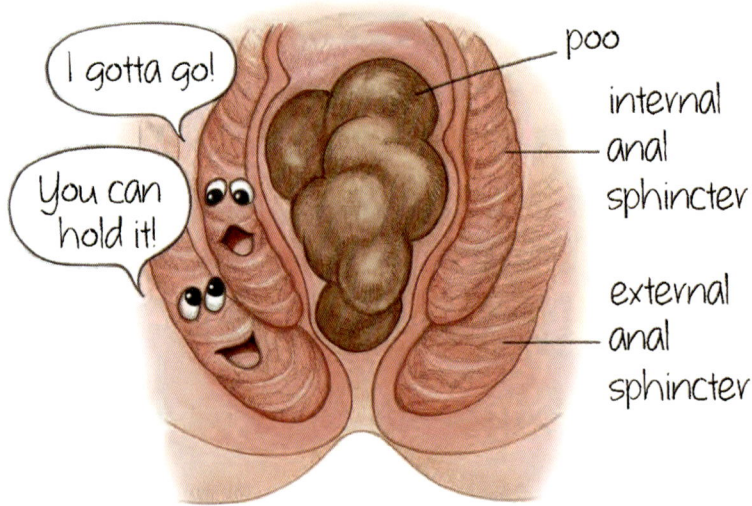

MEET YOUR MICROBIOME

Suppose you consulted a gastroenterologist about the pains in your gut, especially constipation or irregularity. Your gut doctor may surprise you with the first question:

"How's your microbiome?"

"My what?" you may wonder.

If we had to choose one word that would most affect healthy pooing it would "microbiome." Microbiome means "tiny bug home," the name of the community of bacteria that reside primarily in the lining of the large intestine. In return for free food and a warm place to live, they do good things for your body. Think of your gut bugs like the managers of your intestinal health. When explaining this gut-bug home to parents and children, this is what I tell them:

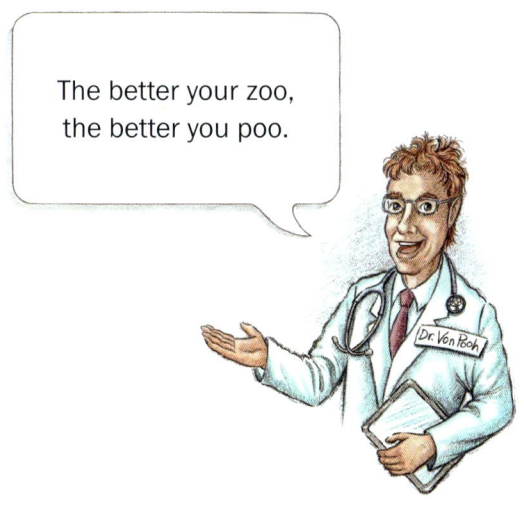

The biggest "zoo" in the world is your microbiome. An estimated 100 trillion bacteria reside in your gut, most of which live in the colon, where more than a billion of these bacteria live in just one drop of intestinal fluid. If you were to bunch all these bugs together in a jar they would weigh around three pounds, making the microbiome one of the largest "organs" in your body. The better these gut bugs digest the fiber you eat, the better is the poop you make.

Your gut pharmacy. We doctors call the microbiome your *internal gut pharmacy* because these good gut bugs take the leftover food that your small intestine couldn't digest, especially fiber, and make medicines out of it. Here's a list of what these good gut bugs do for your body:

- Balance the immune system
- Grow a non-leaky gut lining
- Help prevent allergies
- Ease pains in the gut
- Help keep the body lean
- Make nutrients your body needs
- Defend against harmful bacteria that enter the gut
- Help prevent intestinal "-itis" illnesses
- Lower risk of colorectal cancer
- Mellow your moods

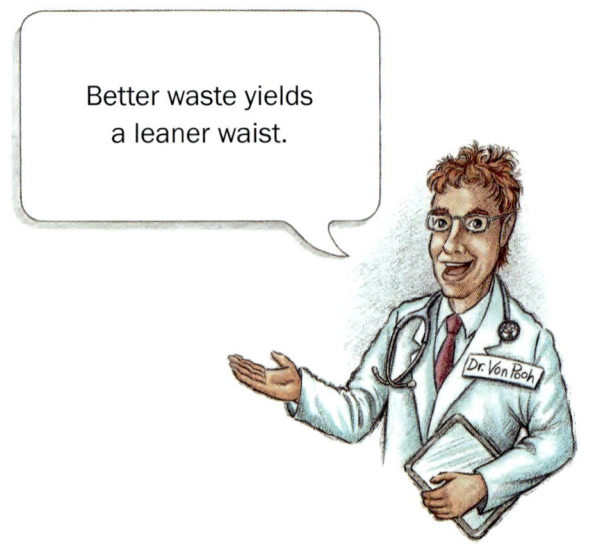

Better waste yields a leaner waist.

MORE ABOUT YOUR MICROBIOME

Microbiome meets immune system. Your microbiome resides in the lining of your gut, in the microvilli, which resembles a shag carpet. It's a beautiful design because not only does it increase the surface area by the many foldings, but all these nooks and crannies form nice little homes and neighborhoods for the resident bacteria to form their own habitat. Picture having your own "bug town" inside your gut.

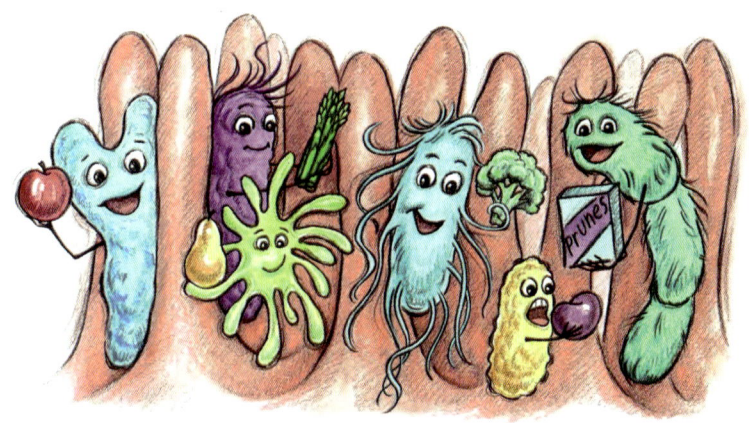

We feed on fiber.

Microbiome digests leftovers. You've heard "eat more fiber," but you're not sure why. The two main reasons are because fiber is the favorite food for your microbiome, and the more fiber-rich your diet, the more comfortable your poop. It's interesting that fiber is a food you can't digest, but your microbiome can. While you may have thought that stringy, chewy stuff on the celery can be unpleasant to eat, it's actually the very food that your gut bacteria thrive on. Think of your microbiome saying, "I'll feed on your leftovers. In return for you feeding me, I'll use these leftovers to fertilize your growing gut garden."

You may hear the term "soluble" and "insoluble" fibers. You need both. A soluble (dissolves in water) fiber is a *prebiotic*, which means it readily ferments into nutrients to feed our friendly flora, which is what the microbiome used to be called, and helps absorb water into the poop. Insoluble fiber is metabolically inert and does not ferment, but it adds bulk to the poop, making bowel movements easier to pass. Good sources of insoluble fiber are grains, nuts, seeds, and the skins of fruits. Think "fiber feeds flora." ("Flora" is the term we use for micro-organisms, the microbiome, in the gut lining because it's like a flower garden.) (Read more about the best fiber for the best pooing, page 43.)

With the modern diet it's almost impossible for us to get our daily requirement of soluble fiber, especially for children. We must be sure to get the full amount and often this means fortifying with the right form of soluble fiber (which we will discuss later). Good sources of soluble fiber are apples, pears, oats, barley, and beans.

Microbiome makes poop. Around half of a healthy evacuation is composed of microbes that have "aged out." They have served their usefulness and "pass out" to make room for younger, healthier microbes. What a smart recycling plant you have keeping you healthy!

Feel good like a gut should. The term "indigestion" is a catch-all term for something uncomfortable happening in the gut. Most of the patients I see for "pains in the gut" have a *messed-up microbiome*. I'll say it again: your poop is a window into your health. When you eat the right fiber-rich foods, your gut bugs can digest the leftover food from the small intestine better. Your microbiome says, "You eat what is good for you; and we'll live off the good-for-us leftovers, and we'll all feel good."

Suppose you consult a top doc in preventive medicine. Let's call her Dr. Good Gut. You open your consultation with, "Doctor, we have so many intestinal problems in our family. I really want to bring up our children to have healthy intestines so they have good gut feelings when they're older. What can we do now to make that happen?"

Dr. Good Gut opens with, "So how's your poop?" Surprised, you wonder why the checkup starts with that usually undercover subject. It's because the healthier the poop, generally the healthier the child. And that's true for all ages.

Dr. Good Gut says, "Have a healthy microbiome. Most of the patients I see at all ages have a messed up microbiome."

Probiotics help you poo. You've probably heard about probiotics, a bunch of good-for-you bugs in a powder. Probiotics (meaning "for life") are billions of good gut bugs that people take to help populate the gut garden with the best bacteria. And, besides probiotics, we need to eat enough good fiber, called *prebiotics*, to feed the good bacteria in our growing gut garden.

The mind-microbe connection. While "my microbiome made me do it" is not totally true, the gut bacteria use the vagus nerve as a superhighway to send messages to the brain, and the brain back to the gut. In some ways the smarter the bacteria in your gut brain, the smarter the tissue in your head brain. Exciting new discoveries reveal that the gut brain and head brain are partners in health. It's fascinating that the gut bacteria can produce neurohormones that alter behavior and emotion and release them into the bloodstream to go to the brain. The head brain and the gut brain have a close relationship. They communicate via biochemical "emails," keeping each other accountable for their actions. If the microbiome is struggling down below, the head brain can develop a bad mood. So instead of your anxiety just being "all in your head," it could also be in your gut. An unhealthy gut can lead to a general feeling of unease, causing a never-ending spiral of internal stress. (See related section, Stress-less Pooping, page 47).

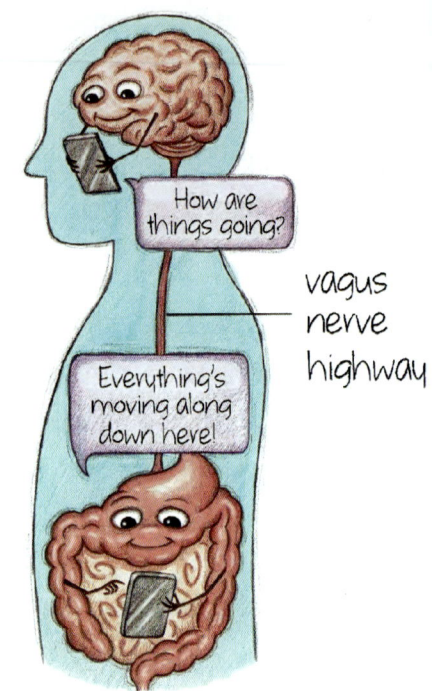

vagus nerve highway

WHAT IS POOP MADE OF?

By now you're wondering what poop is made of. It's half water, and the rest is bacteria, fiber that hasn't been digested, and other kinds of leftovers, such as mucus and intestinal cells that have served their purpose and are being evacuated to make room for new cells. Sixty percent of the dry weight of poop is leftover gut bacteria, much of which have served their usefulness and are passed out, enabling the colon to quickly repopulate with new and healthier ones. Constant repopulation of the gut lining with good bacteria is where our perfect poo program shines.

PORTRAIT OF A PERFECT POOP

Ideally, what should poop look like and what should having a poop feel like? While the portrait of a perfect poop varies among persons at various ages, and even changes weekly within the same person, the healthiest poop should have these characteristics:

Frequency: Preferably three times a day, but at least once a day. For many people who poo perfectly, the number of times they poo equals the number of meals they have.

Consistency: semi-soft, neither golf-ball hard nor watery soft. Dr. Poo helps you firm your poop if too loose, and soften it if too hard.

Color: brown

Feeling: easy to pass without straining

Sinks rather than floats

Good pooping attitude: You have the natural urge to poo and actually look forward to going as opposed to dreading it because it is often painful.

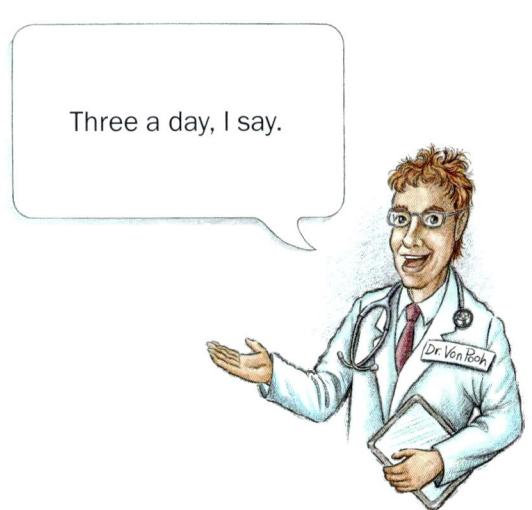

THE TELL-TALE SIGN OF A PERFECT POOP

If the end of the poop tapers to a tail, this usually means your external sphincter (donut muscle) has opened and closed in a more relaxed and less-forced manner. Tail-poop tells you that the size and softness is in the range of perfect poop.

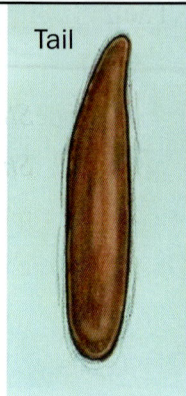
Tail

THE PERFECT POOP PLAN

On page 41 you will learn the Four-Step Perfect Poop Plan. An easy way to remember how what you eat affects how you poo is this: The 2-Ss, *smoothies* and *salads*, produce a 2-S perfect poop:

1. *Slides:* When your poop comes out as one soft, long snake-like piece, around hot dog size, and the resulting anus-to-water distance is so short it doesn't splash, or go "plop," it is probably a near-perfect poop. Yet if it comes out in a few hard, marble-size or even golf ball-size pieces and you hear a "poop plop," and you sometimes feel a tiny watery splash, that's usually a painful "pellet poop." Or, as Dr. Bryce Wylde, author of *Wylde On Health: Your Best Choices In the World of Natural Health*, describes: "Ideally, your poop should enter the toilet bowl as smoothly as an Olympic diver, without a lot of splashes or noise."

2. *Soft:* No golf-ball hardness.

The 2-Ss of painful pooping are:

- *Stuck poop:* See curing constipation, page 53.
- *Shoot poop:* The opposite of stuck poop, it comes out too fast, producing an audible "plop" and it can not only give you a wet bottom, but also irritate the sensitive rectal lining.

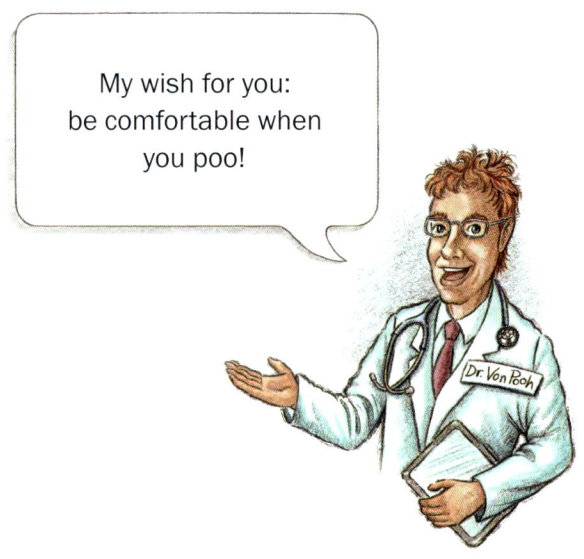

CHAPTER 2
THE THREE-STEP PERFECT POOP PLAN FOR BEGINNER POOPERS: INFANTS AND TODDLERS

Parents, remember our goal: make pooing pleasant for your child, beginning as a newborn. Start baby's life off with the right poop. Follow these three steps to get your precious bundle of joy off to a good start.

STEP 1: FEED BABY THE PERFECT MILK FOR PERFECT POOP

BREASTFEED AS OFTEN AND FOR AS LONG AS YOU CAN

Over my 50 years as a baby-poop observer, I've noticed that most breastfed babies have perfect poop. This observation taught me the most important lesson in perfect pooing:

What children eat affects how they poo.

Feed the right food into the top end and the right poop comes out at the bottom end.

Smell and tell. One huge advantage of exclusive breastfeeding is: poop doesn't smell bad! In our medical practice I can tell what milk a baby is fed by the smell of the leftovers. It might smell and look like honey-mustard, a nice production from your little honey. Poop reveals a lot about a baby's health and nutrition.

Show and tell. Compared to formula-fed infants, the poos of breastfed infants are more frequent, softer, and have an easier-to-pass consistency. Within a couple weeks after birth the poops of healthy breastfed babies usually become yellow, seedy, sweet-smelling, and have a mustard-like consistency. Because breastmilk is a natural laxative, the daily number of poopy diapers is often more for breastfed babies. We often use *stool color change*, from brown to yellow, as a clue that mother's milk has "come in." So, in the early weeks a newborn's stools normally change from brownish-black to greenish-brown to mustard-yellow as baby gets more milk fat. As I examine a baby and take the diaper off, I often say "Good poop! You are feeding your baby good food."

When you feed the microbiome perfect food, it usually produces perfect poop. And it has just been in the past few years that researchers learned why. Moms, are you ready for this? It's called M.O.M. – the term for the microbial mechanism that feeds the microbiome to produce perfect poop. M.O.M. – *m*ilk-*o*riented *m*icrobiota – is technical talk for "Mama's milk makes nutrients her baby's microbiome likes." So, who is the real poop expert? Dr. M.O.M.!

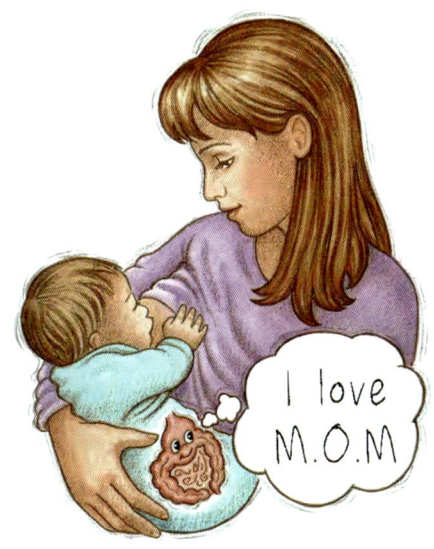

Those mommy-made magic biochemicals are called H.M.O.s – human milk oligosaccharides, special sugars a baby's microbiome loves. So, start baby's gut bugs – and resulting bowel movements – on the right milk.

In fact, once upon a time, before M.O.M. was discovered, formula manufacturers left out H.M.O.s. In 2016, some companies began adding H.M.O.s to infant formula.

Pleasant poopers. Delving deeper into poop psychology, notice the nice smile on a baby's face when they make a poop – no straining, no bloating, no colicky crying – just nice pooping. That's the gut-brain / head-brain connection you want every child to experience: it's pleasant, not painful, to poo.

But life in Diaperville is not always so pleasant. Sometimes it is downright, well, poopy. Some infants and toddlers have more than their fair share of painful poops: constipation and other poopy problems you will learn how to prevent in Chapter 4. If pooping is unpleasant or even painful, toddlers are going to try to avoid pooping or, as moms say, "hold onto it," which only makes the problem worse.

THE SECOND-BEST MILK FOR THE PERFECT BABY POOP

Mothers who for medical reasons are unable to breastfeed completely or even partially, conclude their only choice is to use formula. New insights have downgraded infant formula to the third milk alternative, the second being donor milk.

W.H.O. POO

The long-term health benefits of breastmilk led the *World Health Organization* to advise mothers to breastfeed for at least *two years*. There is a worldwide increase in the use of donor breastmilk. The World Health Organization (WHO) has officially endorsed donor milk as "the second-best milk" for baby.

Designating donor milk as the second-best milk for babies and putting infant formula in third place is one of the newest and poo-healthiest trends in infant feeding. Twenty years ago, this was new. Now it's standard. Breastfeeding friends and relatives are usually delighted to be a "milk donor." Milk banks are sprouting up everywhere. I remember calling the father of one of my milk-needy moms and saying, "How would you like to make the best investment into your new grandson's life?" He was overjoyed at being able to fund the expense for donor milk.

Bottlefeed like you would breastfeed. "Combo moms" (both breast and bottle) would often tell me that their baby poos more often and more comfortably on days when they primarily breastfeed, such as on weekends when they're not working outside the home. When bottlefeeding, there is a tendency to offer baby larger volumes at longer intervals – just the opposite of what the poop-making parts of the gut like. The smaller the volume, the more completely it is digested, and the less leftover there is for the colon to have to process. Some bottlefeeding babies feed in big gulps too fast, and their poo gets out too fast. I learned this by treating "explosive poopers." This nuisance subsided when Mom slowed baby's feedings according to my "rule of twos" – feed baby *half* as much, *twice* as often.

THE SMELL CHANGES AS BABY'S DIET CHANGES

- Formula-fed infants tend to have less frequent, firmer, greener, and smellier poo.
- Combo-feeders (breast and formula) tend to have a combo of both textures and smells.
- Poop smell changes as baby eats solid foods.

STEP 2: BEGIN BABY ON POO-FRIENDLY SOLIDS

Think out of the box. Thankfully, gone are the days when rice cereal was the first solid starter food. Instant rice cereal is not real food—it is too processed. Grains are generally not an intestine-friendly starter food, and they can be constipating. My favorite "poo poem" is from a mom who noticed the real food – real poop connection:

Eat real food
Poop real often
Feel real good.

Dr. Poo thanks you, Kathy Bee

In addition to mother's milk, what food comes close to what baby's head brain and gut brain (the microbiome) need? The first food must have three features:

1. Full of soluble and insoluble *fiber*, a favorite food for baby's growing gut garden.

2. Full of *fat*. Baby's brain is 60% fat. I call them little "fatheads." Mother's milk gets 40-50% of its calories from fat.

3. Mushy and veggie-tasting. Beginning early, you want to *shape young tastes* to crave fiber-rich vegetables.

STARTER FOOD NUMBER ONE: MY TOP PICK FOR BABY'S FIRST FOOD: AVOCADO

Avocado is the fruit highest in healthy fats and protein, the top two "grow-nutrients" that baby needs.

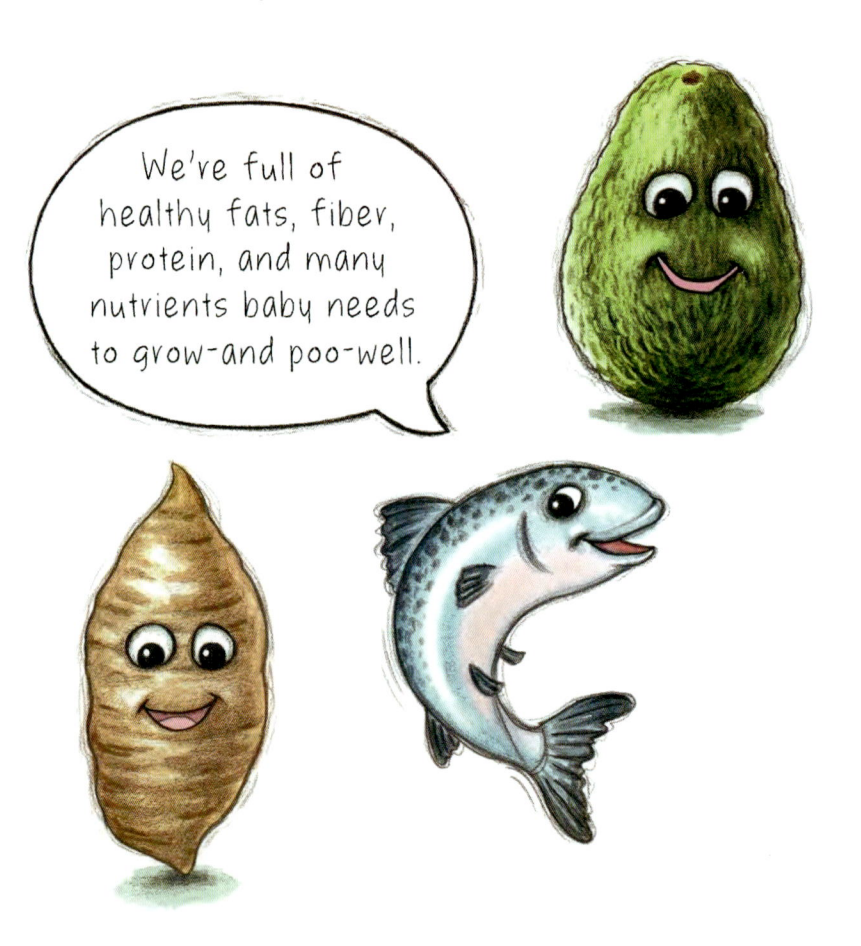

We're full of healthy fats, fiber, protein, and many nutrients baby needs to grow-and poo-well.

STARTER FOOD NUMBER TWO FOR HEALTHY "NUMBER TWO": SWEET POTATOES

They are sweet and fibrous for baby's growing gut garden. Babies are born with a natural preference for sweet tastes. (Mother's milk is naturally sweet.) (For more about choosing solid foods, see AskDrSears.com/StartingSolids)

GO WILD WITH WILD SALMON

Surprised, moms? By a smart design of human development, the top fat in salmon is the top fat in baby's brain. Since a baby's brain doubles in size during the first year, babies need smart foods. Feed fish to your little "fathead." (See more about choosing safe starter seafood: AskDrSears.com/SafeSeafood.)

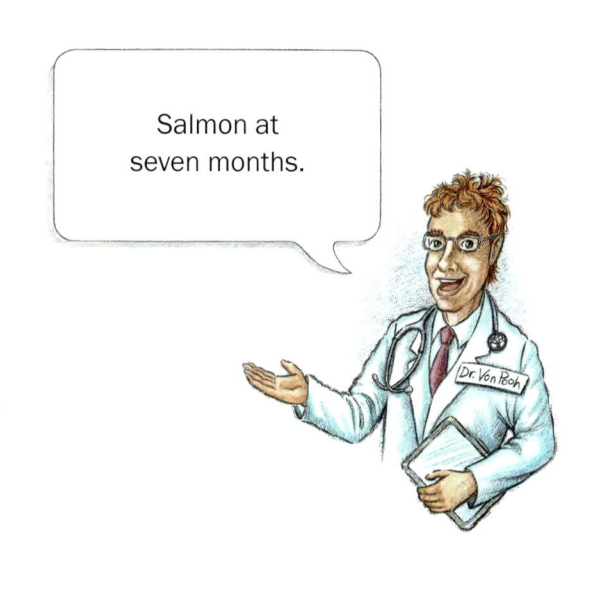

Salmon at seven months.

POO-FRIENDLY FOOD PREPARATION

Think of the consistency of starter foods like the consistency of perfect poop: soft and mushy. Since six to twelve month olds don't have many teeth to "chew-chew times two" (one of the most important lessons in "poopology" that you will learn next), it's important to blend and mash the food. Begin with poo-friendly foods such as avocado, sweet potatoes, bananas, and wild salmon. Babies prefer beginning with *blended* foods (slow speed in a blender), then gradually increase the consistency from blended to mashed. This fits into Adult Poopology 101: the more the top end breaks up the food, the easier it is on the bottom end.

The age at which babies can easily chew and self-mash (called masticate) solids varies from baby to baby. Some sensitive eaters need mushy foods well into the second year.

Poop changes as food changes. Because no solid food is as easy to digest as mama's milk, it's usual to notice a change in poo frequency, color, and consistency with a change in diet. This is why it is so important to continue the volume of breastmilk as you add solid foods. Solids shouldn't replace breastmilk, but, rather, supplement it.

STEP 3: NIBBLE YOUR WAY TO PERFECT POOP

Small, frequent feedings are more likely to yield more frequent, comfortable poops – at all ages. Left to their own devices, toddlers are natural nibblers. They like to pick and eat throughout the day. Remember, toddlers have tiny tummies, around the size of their fist. If they eat too much, too fast, that is a pain in the gut – constipation – waiting to happen.

OUR FEEDING SOLUTION

Prepare a *nibble tray*. Using an ice-cube tray or muffin tin, we put nutritious and delicious tidbits into each compartment, and tagged each fiber-friendly food with cute names: "banana wheels," "broccoli trees," "funny beans."

Since little fingers love to dip, reserve two sections for dips: hummus, organic whole-milk yogurt, guacamole, and goat cheese. Play show-and-tell: "Cheese on trees," as you dip broccoli into cheese sauce.

By the end of the day, the nibble tray will be empty; and your toddler's tummy full. No hassles.

Be Regular!

The simple term "regular" says it all. Your gut, the most sensitive organ in your body, loves being regular, meaning:

- Passing poops that are consistently comfortable and predictable to pass.

- A *regular* number of poos each day, usually at least three.

- Enjoy the after-poo feeling: "I feel so relieved!"

Be regular and enjoy comfortable bowel habits.

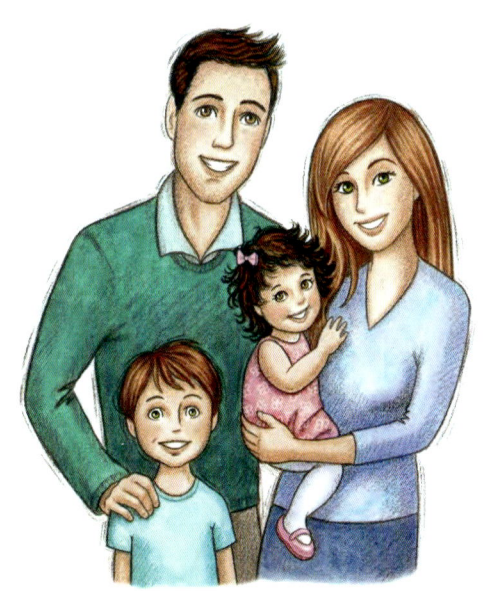

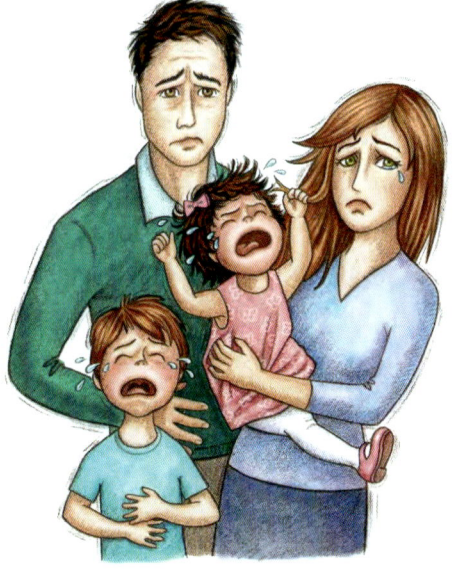

| Happy Poo, Happy Body | Painful Poo, Unhappy Body |

DR. BILL AND MARTHA'S REMEDY FOR BABY CONSTIPATION

Take a bath together. Relax in a tub with warm water breast high. Have someone else hand baby to you. Once baby is also relaxed back-to-chest, massage baby's abdomen.

Massage the movements along. Here's a nice abdominal touch that we have used to ease bloated babies of gas or constipation. We call it the *I Love U* touch of abdominal massage.

1. "I." Place baby on your lap facing away from you, or on the floor nestled on a soft towel. Rub coconut oil in your hands and start massaging using gentle circular motions forming an "I" along Baby's upper left side downward. Imagine you are touch-coaxing any stuck stools to move downward. Oftentimes, this downward left-sided massage is enough to get things moving.

2. "LOVE." Sometimes, if the constipation is worse, gas backs up requiring you to massage across the top of your child's abdomen and down the left side like an upside down "L."

3. "U." If baby is really gassy and bloated, massage the whole abdomen the direction of an upside down "U."

Leg pumping. Another movement to help bowels move poop along is pumping the child's legs in a bicycle motion.

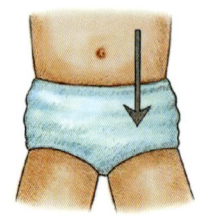

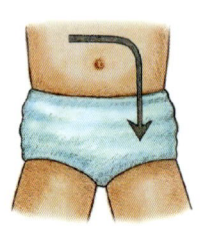

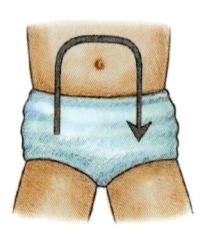

CHAPTER 3
THE FOUR-STEP PERFECT POOP PLAN – FOR ALL AGES

Let's start with the top pooing tip you have already learned:

> When the top end of your G.I. tract enjoys
> better digestion, so does the bottom end.

How and what you eat affects how you poo. With some minor modifications, these tips help all ages poo better, from children to seniors.

STEP 1: CHEW-CHEW TIMES TWO

To help your younger child learn how to poo more comfortably, tell him: "Chew-chew times two" (twice as much as they usually do). For the older child say, "Chew twenty times." Besides releasing more saliva, which is rich in digestive enzymes, chewing slows down your eating so that more digestion can occur in your mouth, and eliminates large amounts of poorly digested food reaching the colon.

Several times a day in my office I prescribe Dr. Bill's "rule of twos":

- Eat *twice* as often.
- Eat *half* as much.
- Chew *twice* as long.

You can do that!

> The more you chew, the better you poo.

If your intestinal tract could talk, it would say: "Grazing is good for me!" Over years of studying the relationship between how people eat and how they poo, I've noticed that fast eaters tend to be painful poopers. That makes sense. The more digestive work you do at the top end, the less wear and tear on the bottom end. Too much poorly digested food arriving in the too fast is a set-up for painful poop.

STEP 2: EAT POO-FRIENDLY FOODS

If you asked your lower intestine what foods it prefers you to eat to have the perfect poop, here's what it would say:

- Foods that are *high* in easily-digested soluble and insoluble fiber, or what we call "fiber-friendly foods."
- *Higher* in plant-based foods, *lower* in animal-based foods.
- Rich in science-based probiotic and prebiotic fiber supplements, especially soluble fiber, which is greatly lacking in our modern diet.
- Food chewed well or blended for easier digestion.
- *Low* in processed foods where the fiber and other rich nutrients have been processed out and artificial ingredients put in.
- *High* in a rainbow of colors – red, green, yellow, purple – from fruits and veggies.

> Eat real foods, enjoy real healthy poop.
> — Dr. Von Pooh

Enjoy a fiber-fluid balance. As you increase the amount of fiber in your diet, you must increase the amount of fluids to keep the balance. As a general guide, for children *an ounce of fluids per pound* of body weight. So, a 30-pound preschooler would need around 30 ounces of fluid. For adults, ½ oz. fluid per pound. Constipation is more common during illnesses because you tend to lose more fluid when you have a fever. So, drink more fluids when sick.

BEST FOODS FOR BETTER BOWELS

The following foods have most of the microbiome and poo-friendly ingredients:

- Apples
- Artichoke
- Asparagus
- Bananas
- Barley
- Beans
- Beets
- Berries
- Broccoli
- Cinnamon
- Cottage cheese
- Endive
- Figs
- Garlic
- Ginger
- Green beans
- Green tea
- Honey, raw (NOT for infants under one year)
- Jicama
- Kale
- Kefir
- Leeks
- Lentils
- Miso
- Oats
- Onions
- Plums
- Pomegranates
- Pears
- Quinoa
- Sauerkraut
- Tempeh
- Tofu
- Vinegar

I have chosen these above foods not only for their high fiber (both soluble and insoluble) and digestibility, but because they are rich in nutrients that feed a healthy microbiome. The better you feed your microbiome, the better you poo. You may notice that most of these foods are "good carbs." Think: good carbs are the ones with good fiber.

Dr. Bill's poo-friendly tip: The two S's, smoothies and salads, tend to be the most poop-friendly. Enjoy a smoothie in the morning and a salad for lunch or dinner, and your gut will thank you.

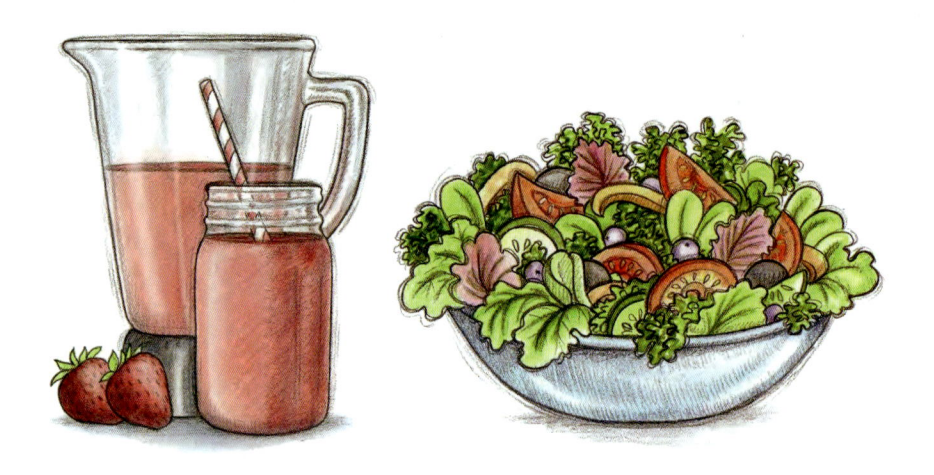

STEP 3: STOOLADE: SHAKE IT OUT – THE TOP TIP FOR POOPING PROBLEMS

The softer your food, the softer your poop. In my medical practice this sipping solution is my top tip for pooing problems.

MY STOOLADE STORY

In 1997, to care for my sick colon, I went through this reasoning:
- Poop that is soft enough and moves through speedily enough is good for you.
- Poop that is hard and moves through sluggishly is bad for you.

I realized that *blending* my breakfast would lead to softer and easier pooing. Wow! What a difference this one simple change made in my pooing comfort. I call my easy-pooing recipe *Stoolade*. (For children with both gut brain and head brain problems I call it *Schoolade.*) It's delicious to drink, and it's the perfect way to supplement with soluble fiber, probiotics, protein, and other nutrients.

> A daily smoothie helps you poo more smoothly.

I have used this one simple tip more than any other in treating patients of all ages with two common "shuns"– indiges*tion* and constipa*tion*. Because the blender does most of the work at the top end, it's easier on the gut to form poop at the bottom end.

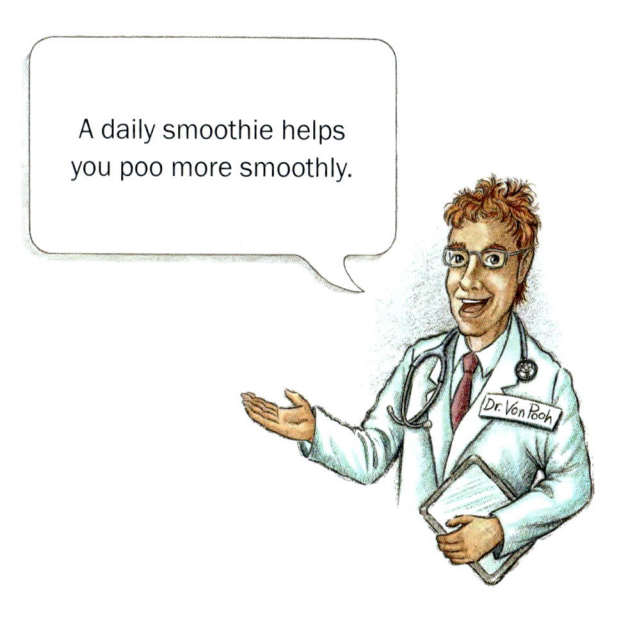

Everybody loves smoothies, especially kids. (See poo-friendly smoothie recipes on AskDrSears.com/smoothies.) The most important poo-friendly foods to add to your daily shake are:

1. *Fiber-rich fruits*: Chopped prunes, plums, pears, pomegranate, figs, banana, apple, avocado, berries, and papaya. Add celery, a handful of kale, spinach or other veggies for a nice green touch. Also, use the skins of plums, pears, and apple, as these are rich in the fiber that is extra poop-friendly. (Add a science-based prebiotic and probiotic fiber supplement, see page 57.)

2. *Fluids*. Your microbiome loves fermented fluids, such as organic kefir. Other fluid options are coconut milk, vegetable juice, and pomegranate juice.

3. *Protein powder.* See AskDrSears.com/SippingSolution

4. *Guar-based soluble fiber.* A scoop of soluble fiber, such as taste-free, grit-free Sunfiber®, enables you to easily add a whopping six grams of gut-friendly soluble fiber per serving. One of the most clinically researched and easy-to-use *prebiotic* soluble fibers, it mixes invisibly without changing the flavor, texture, or aroma.

5. *Special additions:* organic Greek yogurt, nut butters, coconut or hemp oil, ginger, ground flaxseeds or chia seeds, wheat germ, spirulina, shredded coconut, and a prebiotic/probiotic combo such as *Regular Girl*®.

DR. POO ADVISES: BLEND RATHER THAN JUICE

Blending preserves the fiber, which is the top poo-friendly nutrient you want. Juicing usually removes much of the fiber, besides being messy and time-consuming.

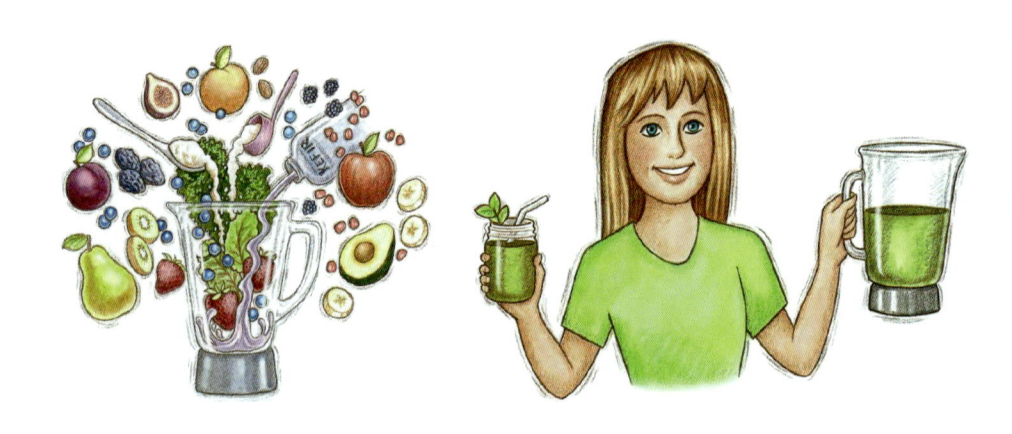

WHICH COUNTRY DO YOU POO IN?

Some cultures poo healthier than others. Cultures that win the Best Poo Award are usually Asians, Indians, and Africans. This is mainly for two reasons: 1) these cultures eat real foods, so they poo right; 2) they eat a high-fiber diet (often three times higher than Americans), so they enjoy easier pooing. Americans, because of the SAD (Standard American Diet), often produce sad poop.

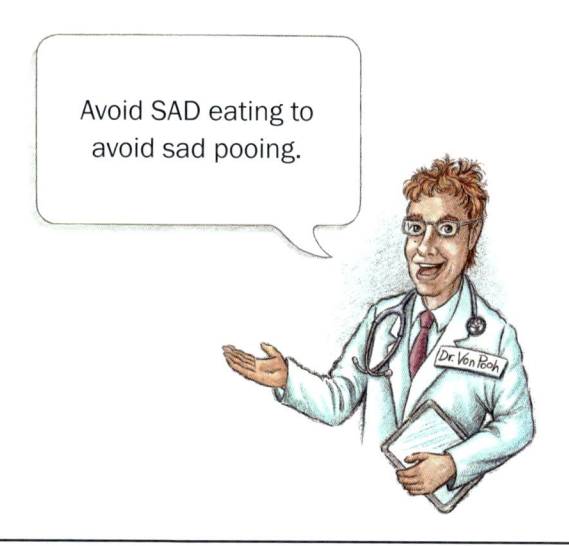

Avoid SAD eating to avoid sad pooing.

STEP 4: DON'T WORRY, JUST POO! STRESS-LESS POOING

As you learned in the mind-microbe section on page 25, how the head-brain feels greatly affects how the gut-brain works. Chronic stress slows digestion and slows bowel motility – two gut problems that lead to constipation and painful pooping. Some chronically stressed persons suffer the opposite – faster bowel contractions leading to diarrhea.

A phrase I use when counselling patients with "leaky gut" is: "You stress, you leak!" Chronic stress damages the sensitive gut lining. (See AskDrSears.com/stressbusters/leakygut).

While stressful thinking is likely to prevent you from pooing properly, there is good news! The organs of the body that are most adaptable to change are the brains – both the head brain and the gut brain. This built-in mechanism of self-repair is called neuroplasticity. Both the brain and the gut say "We're flexible, man! Feed and care for us right and we'll fix the painful poopy problem."

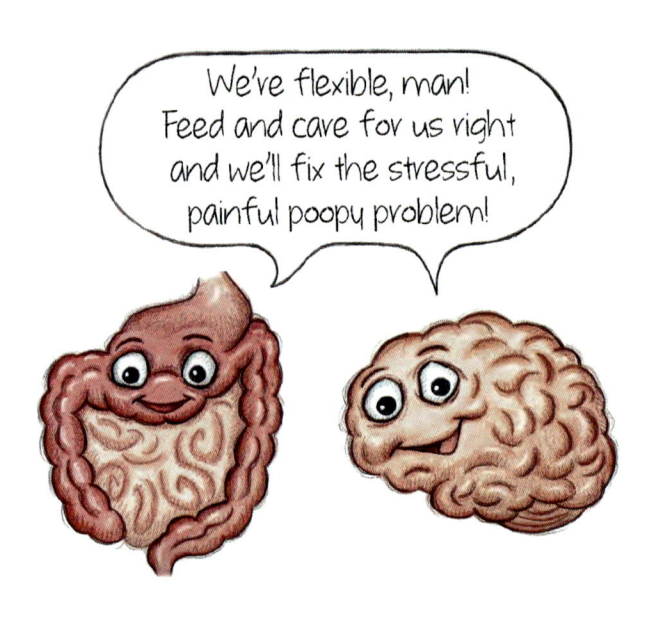

We've flexible, man! Feed and care for us right and we'll fix the stressful, painful poopy problem!

Get ready to digest this mouthful: *psychoneuroendogastroenterology*. This is a new medical specialty that blends brain, gut, and hormonal health together – because all these systems work together. One of the features of a shortened version, *psychoneuroimmunology* (PNI), is how meditation helps the mind to prompt the bowel to "relax and release." It's called *mindfulness-based stool release* (MBSR). (See AskDrSears.com/MBSR).

CHAPTER 4
CURING CONSTIPATION

Constipation tops the list of painful pooping. It's the most common gut pain at all ages, and one I deal with almost daily in my medical practice. The good news: new insights into how to move poop along at just the right speed and the most comfortable consistency can make constipation less of a pain in the gut. Of course it's best to avoid constipation in the first place, if possible, with the prebiotic and probiotic tips already discussed. However, if you do get to this point, here's how to help you poo more comfortably.

MY PELLET POOP STORY

Here's a true confession of how this happened to me: After colon cancer caused me to care more about gut health, I developed my own personal perfect-pooper program. Elimination became so natural, regular, automatic, or whatever you want to call it, that I really didn't think about it much. After all, "poo happens!" You shouldn't have to worry about it, study about it, or make it happen. Then midway through writing this book, I had a painful experience: pellet poop. It was caused by a four-day break in my routine.

The first day was spent on a cross-country plane trip, different diet, different sleep schedule, and different exercise schedule. The first two days I didn't start my day the usual way (meditation, exercise, and smoothie) because my lectures began at 7:30 in the morning. The next two days were full of meetings, lectures, irregular eating, and sitting more than moving. This was the third day I missed my usual morning poos.

I violated the three rules of healthy pooing:

- I *sat* too much. You need to move your body to move our bowels.
- I *ate* constipating meals.
- I let my brain *stress* my gut.

My brain was foggy, my gut was bloated, and I suffered the straining and wear and tear of the worst case of pellet poop I've ever experienced. It's like an inner gut voice, perhaps with some prompts from my microbiome, saying: "You're not living or eating right." I quickly realized that most likely my gut was resenting this sudden change of lifestyle and eating. The gut brain, like the head brain, doesn't like drastic changes, and the painful pellet poops were their protest.

After 24 hours of gnawing pains in the gut and just an overall feeling of "not myself," I spent some time in the gym. Then I went down to the hotel breakfast buffet, gathered up a bunch of fruit, and begged the bartender to blend up my Perfect Pooing smoothie (see page 44), which I sipped on the way to the airport. Upon arrival to the airport I went right to a juice bar, which coincidentally was right next to our departure gate, and got a large create-your-own Perfect Pooing smoothie to sip on the plane. By the end of a day of mental relaxation, gut-friendly eating, and moving my body more, my gut brain and head brain were back to being regular.

Before getting this self-induced pain in the gut, I never fully appreciated what the term "regular" means. "Regular" is just that – normal, automatic, or basically doing what comes naturally. Regularity comes from regularly following gut-healthy habits.

SHOW AND TELL ON-LINE POOP CHARTS

See *DrPoo.com* for downloadable poop charts for all ages. Get used to noticing the character of your poops and what health changes you may need to make.

DR. POO'S SIX-STEP COLON FITNESS PLAN

We're all into "muscle fitness," but I bet there's a group of muscles not on your list to keep fit – the muscles of your colon. How fit is your colon?

Unlike other muscles in your body that wither if you don't "stretch" them, colon muscles don't like to be overstretched.

Problem: Poop that is too large, too hard, and presses against the bowel walls too long causes two problems: the constant pressure of golf-ball poop against the walls of the colon weakens and thins the sensitive lining; it makes its microbiome malfunction.

The muscle-stretching story gets worse. Like a chronically overinflated balloon, pockets of flabby tissue, called *diverticuli*, develop in the weakened colon walls. The hard poop pushes its way into these caves in the walls and gets stuck. A general principle of health is any bodily secretion that gets stuck can get infected – a painful pain in the gut called *diverticulitis*.

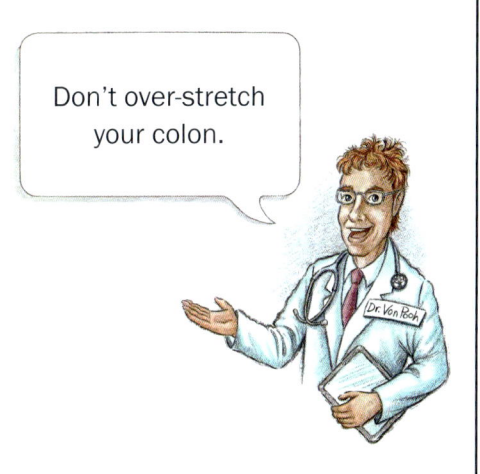

> Don't over-stretch your colon.

Dr. Poo's solution: To prevent diverticulitis, keep your poop semi-soft, frequent, and moving. Remember Dr. Poo's colon fitness plan to keep your poop from getting stuck in your colon:

1. Eat fiber-rich real foods (see list, page 43).
2. Eat according to the rule of twos (see page 41).
3. Enjoy the sipping solution (see page 44).
4. Drink water to your gut's content (see suggested daily volume, page 43).
5. Move your body to move your bowels.
6. Squat smart (see best pooing positions, page 63).

WHY CHRONIC CONSTIPATION IS DANGEROUS

1. Weakens gut muscles. When colon muscles are stretched for weeks, they can weaken, which lessens their pushing power. A painful cycle occurs: the more bowel muscles are stretched, the weaker they become, which worsens constipation and so on. Passing a pellet poop can tear the rectal donut-muscle, causing a rectal fissure (see page 65). It can also cause hemorrhoids. This local rectal wear-and-tear makes it painful to poo. The more it hurts, the more you hold, and the painful cycle worsens.

2. Damages gut lining. Imagine a pile of golf balls constantly pressing against the sensitive gut lining – the "silver lining" that makes so much of the internal medicines you learned about in Meet Your Microbiome (page 21). When these cells are constantly irritated these already rapidly multiplying cells can misbehave and become *cancerous*.

Damaged gut lining can cause *leaky gut*, now a common intestinal problem at all ages.

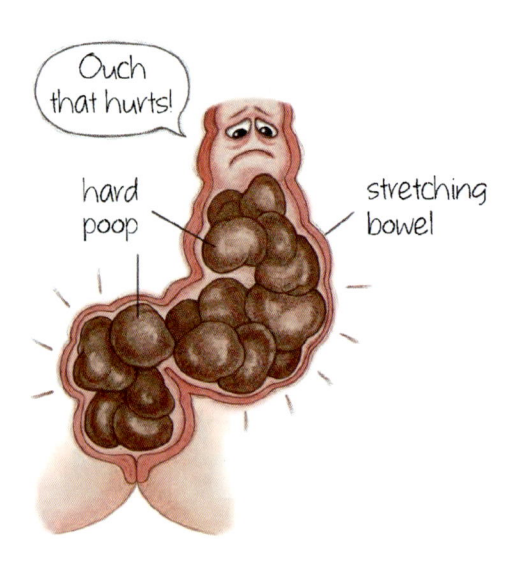

DR. POO'S FIVE-STEP CONSTIPATION CURE

Be patient. Don't worry. The longer that bowel muscles have been stretched and weakened, the longer they may take to heal. It may take six weeks to regain your normal bowel tone, yet it will re-strengthen.

STEP 1: DRINK TO GO

Not drinking enough fluids is a subtle contributor to problems with constipation, especially in the very young and very old. The colon is your body's fluid regulator. If you're not drinking enough, your colon sucks water from the waste material, causing the stool to be water-deprived or hard. People eating high-fiber diets actually increase their risk of constipation if they don't drink extra water along with fiber-rich foods, since fiber needs water to do its intestinal sweeping job. Having more fluids in your diet puts more fluids in your bowels, lessening constipation. As a general guide for adults, drink at least ½ ounce of fluid per pound of body weight. So, if you weigh 150 lbs., you need at least 75 ounces of fluids per day. Many children need one ounce per pound.

STEP 2: ENJOY THE SIPPING SOLUTION

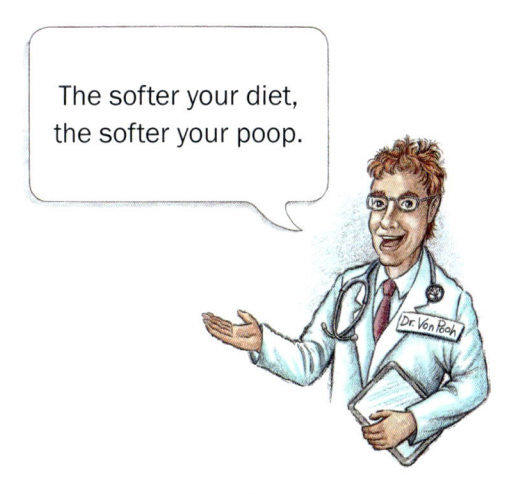

> The softer your diet, the softer your poop.

STEP 3: GET MOVING

A moving body moves the bowels. Besides improving digestion, exercise speeds stool passage through the intestines.

STEP 4: EAT MORE POO-FRIENDLY FOODS

Especially poo-producing are the four P's: Pears, prunes, plums, and peaches.

STEP 5: ENJOY MORE DAILY FIBER

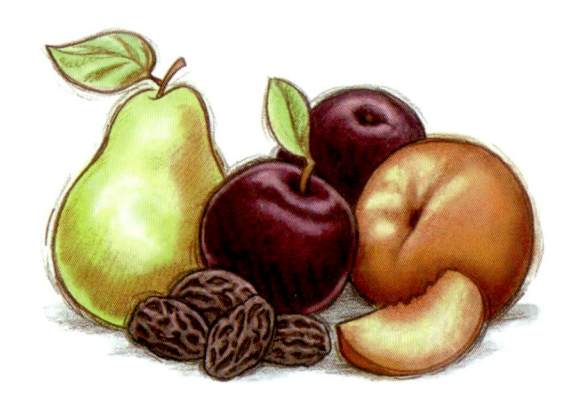

DR. POO'S RECOMMENDED DAILY FIBER – FOR ALL AGES

Infants and Children: Age plus 10 grams. For example, a five-year-old should get 15 grams of fiber daily.

Adults: At least 30 to 40 grams daily

The earliest eating-pooing correlation I noticed was the more daily fiber I ate, the fuller I felt sooner into a meal. That curbed my urge to overeat. Next, I noticed the more fiber I ate, the more frequent and comfortably I pooed. These good-gut feelings prompted me to continue eating an average of *50-60 grams* of fiber daily – around four times the national average of people in our constipated country.

IN SEARCH OF THE PERFECT FIBER SUPPLEMENT

Besides the fiber-rich and gut-friendly foods listed on page 43, sometimes it helps to move things along by adding a fiber supplement, especially a prebiotic soluble fiber. Remember supplements are just that – in *addition* to a fiber-friendly diet, not *instead* of.

A fiber-rich diet contains two types of fiber. Both are necessary for good-gut health. *Insoluble* fiber acts like an intestinal broom to push stuff along. *Soluble* fiber acts like a sponge to absorb water and a prebiotic to nourish your microbiome, or good-gut bugs.

I'm a show-me-the-science doctor. So, I researched medical journals in search of the best science-based fiber supplements. A gut-friendly fiber supplement should have the following qualities:

1. **Slowly draws water into the poop.** Isn't that what you want to do? Like a natural water-loving magnet (scientifically called *hydrophilic*, or water-loving), the fiber slowly – emphasis on *slowly* – softens the stool by increasing its water content. If the fiber works too fast, you could feel bloating and have too-loose poop. A slo-mo fiber is just what Dr. Poo orders.

2. **Plant-based fiber.** During my upgrade to being a nutrition-based parent and doctor, I learned to trust nutrients that naturally occur in plants. I don't trust fiber that is fabricated in a lab.

3. **Feeds your microbiome with a prebiotic.** In the past, fiber was incorrectly labeled "indigestible," which was interpreted to mean it just passes right through your bowels, softens stools, and does

nothing else good for the gut. This fiber-fallacy is only half-true. Yes, your gut doesn't "digest" that chewy fibrous asparagus stalk, but your microbiome does. In science-based writings about fiber, you won't read the term "indigestible" anymore.

The best plant-based fibers act as a "prebiotic," or food for your "probiotics" – your gut bugs. They deliver true regularity without leading to constipation or diarrhea. Unfortunately, many so-called fibers often only help with constipation and not "regularity." Many lead to excess gas, bloating, loose stools, and worse, the dreaded diarrhea. (See more about how your microbiome digests leftovers, page 23.)

4. **Good taste.** Infants, children, and all ages, just won't continue with enough of the fiber supplement if it has an unpleasant taste or texture.

5. **Ferments slowly in your colon.** The right fiber for the right poo must *slowly* ferment, just fast enough to make those internal medicines you learned about on page 22, but not so fast to bloat you from too much gas. *Inulin*, for example, is included in many of the fiber-rich foods and supplements on the market today, but for many it can lead to unpleasant gas, bloating and loose stools.

6. **Gluten-free.** For fiber-conscious consumers, "gluten free" is the new seal of approval. While not always necessary, nor science-based, gluten-free foods are more trusted. Why? Because we no longer grow *real* wheat. It is genetically-modified and toxin-sprayed. The real wheat I grew up with is now a rarity. And American guts are protesting.

Eating a gluten-free diet is easier than ever thanks to the wide assortment of gluten-free products entering the market. Yet, many gluten-free products are low in fiber. Look for breads made with bean or nut flours, and add more high-fiber foods to your diet, such as vegetables and seeds. Because it's tough to consistently get enough fiber, consider a natural fiber supplement like Sunfiber® or Regular Girl®.

7. **Normalize transit time and gut pressure.** The longer food stays in the gut, the more it is likely to cause constipation and pressure against the sensitive gut lining – a double whammy against good gut health. Let's call transit time the *poo-emptying time,* like a train travelling through the tunnel-like intestines. Here's a tip from Dr. Bryce Wylde: to test the transit time in you or your child, try the *beet test*. Chew a handful of cooked, diced beets, usually with the evening meal, then record the time you notice the next reddish tinge to your poop. Repeat this three times to calculate the average transit time. Ideally, the transit time should be from 18-24 hours. If longer, do Dr. Poo's Four-Step Perfect Poop Plan on page 41. After a week, re-test the transit time. You should notice that it shortens. If so, say thank you, Dr. Poo.

FIBER SUPPLEMENTS SUPPORTED BY SCIENCE

Because it's tough to consistently get enough fiber, consider a natural fiber supplement like Sunfiber® or Regular Girl®, the only gluten-free, non-GMO, slowly fermenting and truly regulating fibers on the market. In my quest for the most science-based fiber to use in my medical practice, I realized that guar-gum in general and Sunfiber® in particular is highly studied. It is truly regulating and enjoys all seven of the qualities of the right fiber for the right poo.

1. Science-based.
2. Plant-based
3. Slow, steady water absorbing
4. Slow fermentation to avoid bloating
5. Prebiotic to feed the microbiome
6. Promotes more physiologic poo-emptying time
7. Gluten free and taste ok; a bland taste so kids may not detect it.

Sunfiber® is backed by more than 100 published studies related to IBS, glycemic index, reduction of cholesterol, regulating constipation and diarrhea, satiety, childhood abdominal pain, inflammation, diabetes, and much more. Sunfiber® had its health claims approved and awarded a recommendation from the Canadian Government (Health Canada) to help issues related to IBS and childhood constipation (until now the only recommendation was to take prune juice!). When the U.S. FDA revised the nutrition labeling and fiber definition in May 2016, they specifically identified guar fiber as the only low viscosity (no thick, gloppy mess) soluble fiber having a beneficial physiological effect to human health as a dietary fiber.

For more about selecting science-based fiber supplements, see AskDrSears.com/FiberSupplements where you can download links to where to get the best science-based fiber supplements and how much to take for the good-gut feelings you wish to have.

CHAPTER 5
ASK DR. POO: MORE QUESTIONS YOU MAY HAVE

I've compiled frequent concerns I address in my medical practice. For more poo topics, see our website: DrPoo.com

POO AT SCHOOL
My child got so constipated when starting school. Why?

This is often the start of a lifelong issue of the socially embarrassing relationship between their gut and poop. Kids love talking about, thinking about, and looking at their poop. Our society teaches them that this is a bad thing that should be avoided and that is embarrassing. Get over it! Teach them to be comfortable with all their natural bodily functions.

Poo anxiety, poo-withholding, constipation, or whatever you want to call this painful practice is particularly common when children go off to school. They leave their favorite pooing place (their home bathroom) and are forced to poo in a strange bathroom. Coupled with an often poo-unfriendly diet and beginning school stress, the beginning pooper and schooler becomes a setup for potty anxiety. Starting school sets up children for constipation. They are too busy to poo during play, too afraid to poo during school, and too pooped to poo when tired or drained.

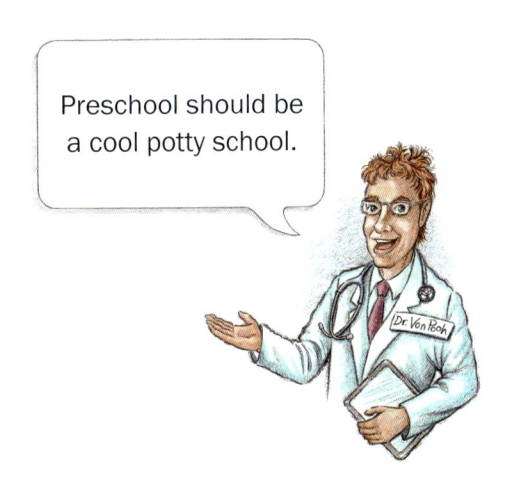

> Preschool should be a cool potty school.

First day of school. While bathroom checks are not high on the list of interviewing perspective preschools, it's worth a trip to see if it's a fun place to poo: cute toddler-friendly pictures on the wall, toddler-size toilets—any child-centered décor that prompts an anxious toddler that this is a fun place to poo. After all, the reason you send your children off to school in the first place is to teach them tools to succeed in life. Perfect pooing is one of those tools.

HOLDING POO

My three-year-old holds onto his poop. He sometimes refuses to go and I just know he needs to by the look on his face and how he's squatting. Is this hurting him?

Yes. Not listening and following through on your gut signals is bad for the bowels. Let's look at what's going on in there to understand what happens when you stubbornly don't listen to this automatic self-evacuation system. At the lower end of the colon just above the anus are two donut-like muscles called sphincters. The inner one, called the internal sphincter, is just on top of the outer one, or the external donut muscle, the one you see when you insert a suppository or wipe the child's bottom.

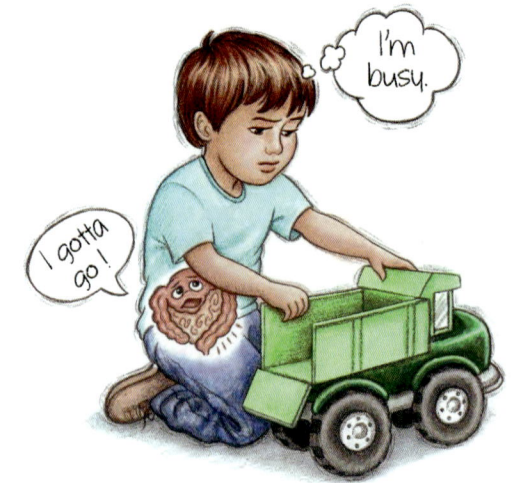

These two donut muscles are partners in pooing. The internal one is connected by a nerve pathway to the brain. When that internal donut muscle gets stretched because poop is pressing on it, it sends a message up to the brain – call it a poo prompt – that tells the child: "Hey, you're full down there, go poo." This automatic feedback-evacuation system is not really under the child's control. Yet, it's not always possible, nor socially acceptable, to poop every time the brain says so. So the second muscle, the external donut muscle, is under your conscious control. You can squeeze it and hold onto the poop and eventually overrule your brain/internal donut muscle connection. This muscle-signaling override is particularly common in young children who may be too busy to poo, too embarrassed to poo (such as in preschool), or just plain don't want to.

Two problems occur when this mental and physical evacuation system is not followed. First, when the head brain / gut brain communication system is not listened to, the head brain eventually concludes, "That stubborn gut-brain muscle down there isn't listening to me when I tell it to evacuate, so I'm just going to take a vacation and quit yelling at it. Eventually, it will learn to listen to me." Secondly, we have a muscle-stretching problem. The internal donut muscle stretches, gets weakened, the poop backs up, and the whole lower colon muscle stretches and weakens, just the opposite of what you want to push poop out. In fact, when I examine a child with a history of severe constipation, I can often feel "a bunch of golf balls" in the lower left abdomen.

Eventually, this becomes a painful cycle. The longer he holds onto the poop, the more painful it is to poo, which causes him to hold onto it, and the weaker everything gets. Occasionally, colon muscle will squirt a bit of loose poop around the golf balls and out the bottom, soiling underwear, which may be mistaken by mom as diarrhea. In fact, when I diagnose constipation, mothers are often surprised that the loose, watery squirts are a clue to constipation. One of the best psychological terms I have heard for what I simply call stopping poop-holding is *defecatory discipline*.

DR. POO'S THREE-STEP METHOD TO RELEASE STALLED STOOL

1. **Read and do Chapter 4,** Curing Constipation.

2. **Play show and tell.** Using the diagram to the right, show your child what happens when he holds in his poop. Emphasize good-gut feelings: "You'll feel so much better and have less tummy-aches when you poo three times a day."

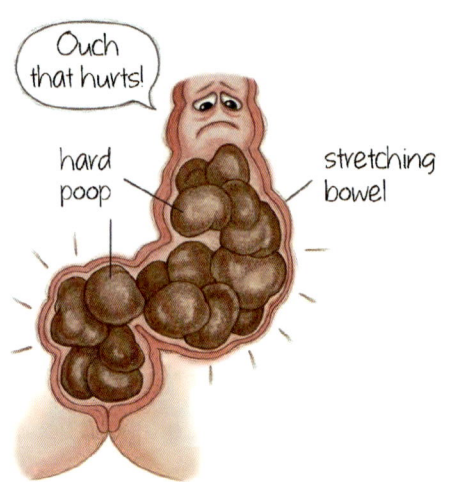

   Ouch that hurts!

   hard poop — stretching bowel

3. **Have a poo chart.** Similar to a "dry-night" chart for bedwetters, keep a log of when he poos. Perhaps even reward the three poos a day.

   View our poo video on DrPoo.com. We show your child the ouchy stretching of the donut muscles and the pains in the gut that happen when you don't poo properly.

FEAR OF FLUSHING
Our three-year-old hates to flush his poop. Should I be concerned?

Some kids have a fear of flushing, and others laugh at it. While some toddlers just can't fathom flushing part of themselves down the hole, others get sort of a kick out of it: "I pooped, I flushed, and bye-bye mess." If your child has this flushing fear, accept it as a passing quirk of body-sensitive childhood. Like most early pooping problems, it soon will pass.

BEST POOPING POSITION

My five year old sometimes has a hard time, shall we say, getting it all out. How can I help him?

How you sit can greatly affect how comfortably you poop. Moms, pardon the analogy, but a lot of comfortable pooping lessons were learned by watching how veteran "natural childbirthers" squat during delivery.

I never thought about pooing positions until going to Japan. In fact, high on my wish list is a Toto toilet with all those great squirty gizmos. But when nature called when I was out and about in public places in Japan, I had to get accustomed to the toilet-less stall where you just hold onto a side bar and squat over a hole in the floor. No Toto. I noticed that while I missed the niceties of the Toto, my poop came out easier when I squatted, knees slightly higher than bottom. Again, pardon the analogy, but I had seen so many women use the same position during childbirth that I thought this may be the natural way to relax those pelvic floor openings. The reason seems to be that the squatting position straightens out the colon so that it is less curved, giving the poop a straighter shot out with less effort.

I discovered a study done in Japan where they fed volunteers a substance that let their poop show up on x-rays. They found that squatting straightens out the poop tunnel. They also concluded that the exit-protecting donut muscle, called the *levator ani*, relaxed better in the squatting position.

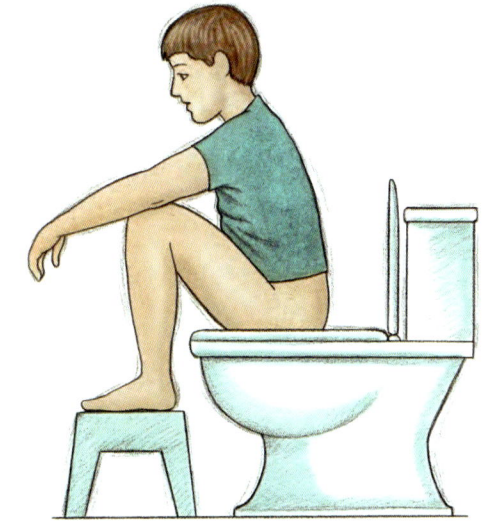

Pushing your feet against a stool helps push the poop out. After learning that, I went to the garage and got out our old nursing stool and now call it my "squat stool." Place the stool in front of the toilet, put your feet on it, elevate your knees at least several inches above your bottom, and you're in the squat position to make it easier to go.

DANGLE POOING

Our three year old likes to sit on our toilet, and it's kind of cute. Is this okay?

If he poos comfortably, it's fine. Yet, I call this "dangle pooing." When the feet dangle from the toilet seat, especially if the knees are lower than the bottom, that position curves the rectal passage and tightens the rectal muscles, making it more difficult to push out the poop. Try putting a stool or box underneath your child's feet to elevate his knees a few inches above his bottom and ask him if he poos better in that position. This is also one of the reasons why low child-size toilets are usually more user-friendly to a child's little body. Children are in a natural squat position on toilets that are made for their size. We have a toddler potty next to our adult potty in our medical office. Parents are surprised when I point out the difference in the child's position when he squats on his own pot.

TELL-TALE UNDERWEAR

I've noticed watery squirts of stool on my child's underwear. Could he have diarrhea?

Just the opposite. He probably suffers from *constipation*. Surprised? This is called "fecal soiling" or "fecal incontinence." Your child is likely so stuffed up with stool that the colon muscles push fluid fecal matter past the obstruction and into the underwear. Because the colonic muscles are so stretched, the nerves don't sense the problem, causing your child to leak without even realizing it. Soiling, and constipation, is more common in boys who notoriously ignore their internal "go-poo" prompts. When I examine a child with tell-tale underwear, I often feel what I call the *golf ball sign*—masses of hard poop in the lower left abdomen. This finding surprises mom when I diagnose, "Your child is severely constipated."

This is really a call to action, or in this case, movement.

1. Go through the Curing Constipation steps in chapter 4.
2. With guidance from your healthcare provider, use a rectal suppository (see recommendations on DrPoo.com) to lubricate the tissues.
3. Your healthcare provider may recommend an enema to disimpact the backed-up bowel mess, even get stuff moving quickly. Oftentimes, after a quick clean-out the child feels so much better that he is likely to pay more attention to his natural poo prompts.

BLOOD STREAKS IN POO
I've noticed a few red streaks of blood in the poo in her diaper. Should I be concerned?

Probably not. Yet when observing any blood in poop at any age, follow the safety principle: when in doubt, check it out. Called a *rectal fissure*, this common and usually self-correcting quirk occurs in the first few months when babies are learning how to poo properly. One hard poop, one hard strain, and *rip* goes the sensitive rectal lining and baby has a tear in the rear.

Take this as a clue to review baby's feeding and pooing patterns (see page 37). Your healthcare provider, after examining the fissure, may recommend using a glycerin suppository (see page 73) with every straining poop for a few days to help the fissure heal.

BLOOD IN POOP? MUST SEE YOUR DOCTOR!

Any blood of any color at any age is a must-see your doctor, especially persistently black "tarry" stools.

STINKY POO

Sometimes my child's poo smells awful, other times it's ok. Why?

I call this the "smell and tell" sign that a change in eating habits causes a change in odor. The longer intestinal contents hang around inside, the more they stink, for several reasons. The microbiome, those hard-working gut bugs you learned about on page 21, are producing smelly, gaseous by-products, such as hydrogen sulfide. The longer poop stays in, the more it smells, because those bugs start working overtime and they're not happy about it. It's their way of protesting. While perhaps not always true, poopologists believe that eating meat produces more of a stink than eating plants. This makes sense since the microbiome prefers to digest plant-based foods. You can probably correlate his smelly poops with what he had for dinner the day before.

To help his poop be more socially acceptable, teach your child to follow the perfect pooing plan on page 51. As so many nuisances of childhood do, this problem will pass and he will eventually have more pleasant poop.

TWEEN POO
How do I talk with my pre-teen about healthy bowel habits?

Parents talk with their children about the birds and bees, and watching out for strangers, and moms with their daughters about their menstrual cycle. Poop is an often overlooked subject but just as important because it is a window to how healthy we are. Knowing that your child understands this will give you both peace of mind.

Start by using the Dr. Poo chart at the end of this book to show what normal, healthy poop should look like. Ideally, a child should go about 3 times a day, with poop similar to type 3 or 4 on the chart.

Specifically for your daughter: if she needs to improve her poop shape, increasing her intake of prebiotic fiber and probiotics can help. Regular Girl® makes fun on-the-go stick packs which contain both fiber and probiotics. She can easily slip a pack into her purse, backpack, or pocket. Just sprinkle one serving into her favorite non-carbonated cold beverage or food and the comfort of a regular day is hers. She won't taste the difference, but she'll feel the benefits.

Our twelve-year-old is starting to get early acne. I've heard this could be related to pooing patterns?

Right! I call this the a*cne-constipation connection.* Best way to clear the skin is to clean out the gut. There is a gut-brain / skin relationship. Gut doctors who studied adolescents are finding, not surprisingly since the brain and the skin are derived from the same embryologic cellular roots, that what's good for the head brain is good for the skin. Science agrees. A clue came when gut doctors found that adolescents with the most acne were also those who had the most problems with gut pains. Their conclusion was that since acne is a form of skin inflammation and the microbiome helps balance inflammation that this is the basic mechanism: the better your microbiome, the better the skin. This is important because it may be one way to get "how-do-I-look" teens, and even tweens, to pay attention to how they feed their gut in addition to what they put on their skin. Doctors have long known that the better you care for your gut, the better your skin looks. Studies have shown that adolescents who eat more junk food – especially fast food that's sweetened, fried, and low in nutrient density – may have worse acne.

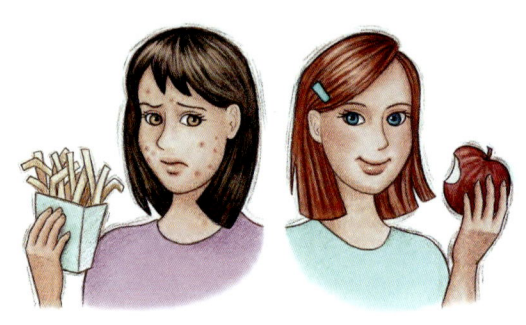

The gut-skin mechanism seems to be that stress plus a junk-food diet (which is mainly low fiber) slows gut motility and weakens the microbiome, resulting in a decrease in normal microbial biofilm (the microbiome-rich film on the intestinal lining), especially the most intestinal-protective gut bug, *bifidobacteria,* which I dub BIF. This leads to intestinal permeability, or leaky gut, allowing endotoxins to get into the bloodstream, and into the skin. Psychological stress also slows small intestinal transit time, encouraging overgrowth of harmful bacteria and compromising the intestinal barrier. (See AskDrSears.com/DrPoo/ScientificReferences for the Sunfiber® acne study.)

POOPING WHILE PREGNANT
I'm seven months pregnant and getting more constipated. Help!

That baby bump you see getting bigger is also putting pressure on your intestines. Pregnancy constipation is your gut's way of telling you, "It's getting crowded in here."

Four Ways to Constipation Relief During Pregnancy:

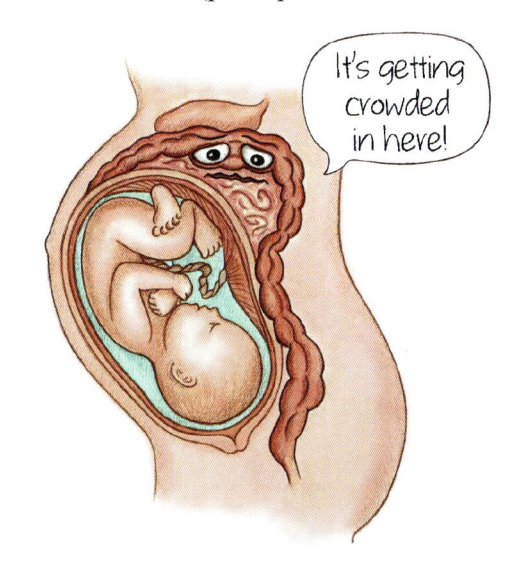

Most women are prone to constipation throughout their pregnancy. Early in pregnancy you can again blame pregnancy hormones, which slow the movement of food through your intestines. In physiologic jargon, this change is called decreased gastrointestinal motility. The slower passage of food and fluid allows more fluid to be absorbed (perhaps another one of nature's ways of ensuring that you get the necessary fluids into your system). The combination of reduced motility of the intestines and firmer waste products (since more fluid has been absorbed) contributes to constipation. In later pregnancy, the pressure of your enlarging uterus on the large intestine further hinders the passage of stools. The good news is you can outwit this uncomfortable effect of your hormones by eating foods that increase the water content of your bowel movements and foods that naturally travel faster through your intestines. Try these tips for constipation relief during pregnancy:

1. *Enjoy Stoolade*, a perfect way to eat for good gut feelings (see page 44).
2. *Do the rule of twos* – grazing (page 41).
3. Enjoy poo-friendly foods (page 43).
4. Take a daily fiber supplement that is safe for mom and baby (see RegularGirl.com)

GREEN POOP
Sometimes my baby's poop is green. Should I worry?

Poop starts out green, yet as it moves through the curvy intestinal highway the body reclaims much of its green bile – an efficient recycling system. Poop gradually goes from dark green, to light green, to brown. Most of the color you see is due to the time it takes for the poop to make its way from the beginning of the intestines to the end. If it moves through quickly, it's going to come out greener. If it goes slow, most of the green bile will be absorbed by the time it exits. Several times a week I reassure parents who are worried that an occasional green poop in an otherwise healthy, comfortable baby is usual and a non-worry.

GASSY POO
When I'm constipated I also pass more gas. Why?

The same microbial mechanism that makes poop makes gas. The term for how your gut makes gas is "fermentation." If bacteria couldn't produce gas, a by-product of metabolism, we wouldn't have some favorite foods like kefir, yogurt, wine, cheese, vinegar, miso, and many others.

When the gut bugs work fast, they produce less gas. Yet, if the poop lingers too long, say intestinal transit time gets slow, the bacteria have more time to produce gas. That's why the formula for good gut health, and less gut smell, is: chew it, digest it, move it quickly along, ferment it and pass it. This leaves less time for extra gas. Think of your intestinal contents: "pass fast, less gas."

MORNING POO
Why is my poop harder in the morning?

During the day, you move things along and out because you are moving your body and drinking more fluid. While you are sleeping, everything slows and fluid intake lessens. This slowed intestinal pace hardens poop. Try these poo tips:

1. Enjoy a before-bed poo-friendly snack. By eating poo-friendly food in the evening, you are more likely to enjoy a more pleasant morning poo.

2. Drink more water in the evening before retiring, unless, of course, that makes you get up more to pee.

3. Sip eight ounces of your leftover poo-softening shake as your bedtime snack. Let your gut bugs enjoy feasting on their favorite food during the night. Perhaps they will thank you with a softer morning poo.

PRE-OP POO

My son is going to the hospital for surgery. I've heard that anesthesia often causes constipation. How can we help him?

Anesthesia does slow gut motility, and so does post-op medication. You are on the right track to plan ahead.

Stoolade to the rescue. Every day for at least three days before surgery, serve your child his favorite smoothie (see page 44). Then after surgery, let him sip on a shake all day long once you get clearance from the medical staff. In our local hospital, the nurses say, "Oh, it must be one of Dr. Sears' patients – we hear the blender going." As one of my patients put it: *"My smoothie is my soothie!"*

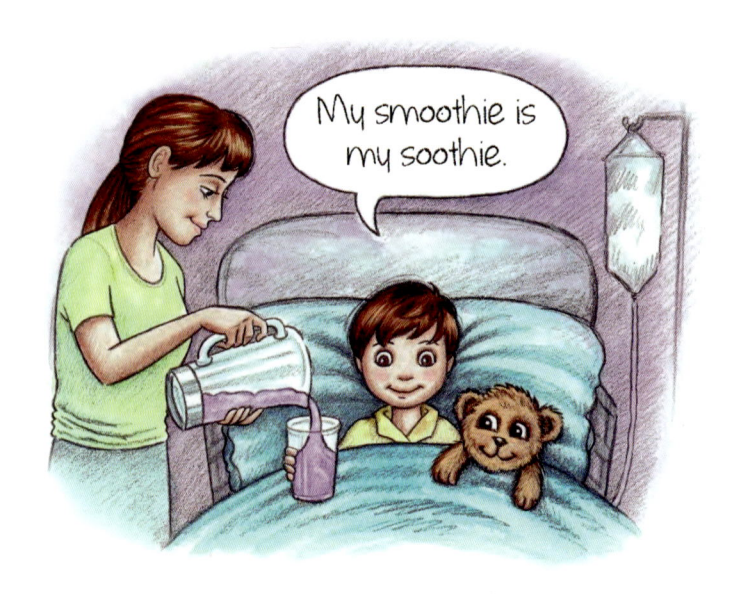

NATURAL LAXATIVES

Our family has a lot of constipation problems. What can I get at the pharmacy to help?

Glycerin suppositories. Available without a prescription, they look like one-inch rocket ships. They are very useful for the straining, stopped-up baby or toddler.

- As soon as you see the "gotta-go" straining signs of "I'm trying to go but can't," lay baby on the floor as you would while changing a diaper.

- Insert the suppository into the rectum then hold the buttocks together for a few minutes to allow the glycerin to dissolve and lubricate the lower colon and soften the stool. As you insert the suppository, wiggle it a bit to stimulate and relax the tense rectal muscles.

- Sing fun songs with cute facial antics just for this occasion. Baby will laugh and relax – and poo!

GIVE YOUR FAMILY AN OIL CHANGE

Flax oil is our family's favorite. If you're going to "oil" the bowels, consume one that has some nutritional value. That where flax oil shines as a rich source of healthy omega fats.

Infants: one teaspoon a day
Toddlers: two teaspoons a day
Children and adults (who think they're kids ☺): one tablespoon a day

Flaxseed, ground, is even better because it is fiber-rich. Grind your own, ten seconds in a coffee grinder. Put one tablespoon for children or two for adults into the stoolade smoothie.

NO-NO TO MINERAL OIL
Besides having no nutritional value, mineral oil is a petroleum byproduct, and if overused can lessen absorption of vitamins and minerals.

Olive oil. Drizzle two to three teaspoons of extra virgin, cold-pressed olive oil on the evening salad. One of the most nutritious oils, besides softening stools, olive oil shapes a child's tastes toward liking oils that are good for the gut.

Psyllium Husks. Fine flakes of psyllium bran are a family favorite. Begin with a teaspoon a day added to a smoothie and gradually increase to two teaspoons a day. Yet, for a better taste and more mouth-friendly texture, instead of the thick, gloppy psyllium, add a scoop of taste-free, glop- and grit-free Sunfiber® or Regular Girl® to anything, even water or juice may be the way to go.

ENJOY A FIBER-FLUID BALANCE

When adding ground flax or psyllium to your daily diet, make sure to increase your fluid intake as well. An easy fluid rule to remember: for each added teaspoon of fiber, drink two extra 8-ounce glasses of water. Otherwise, fiber without fluid equals gummed-up poop. However, this is not really an issue with a low viscosity soluble fiber like Sunfiber®. It's only an issue for high viscosity fibers like psyllium.

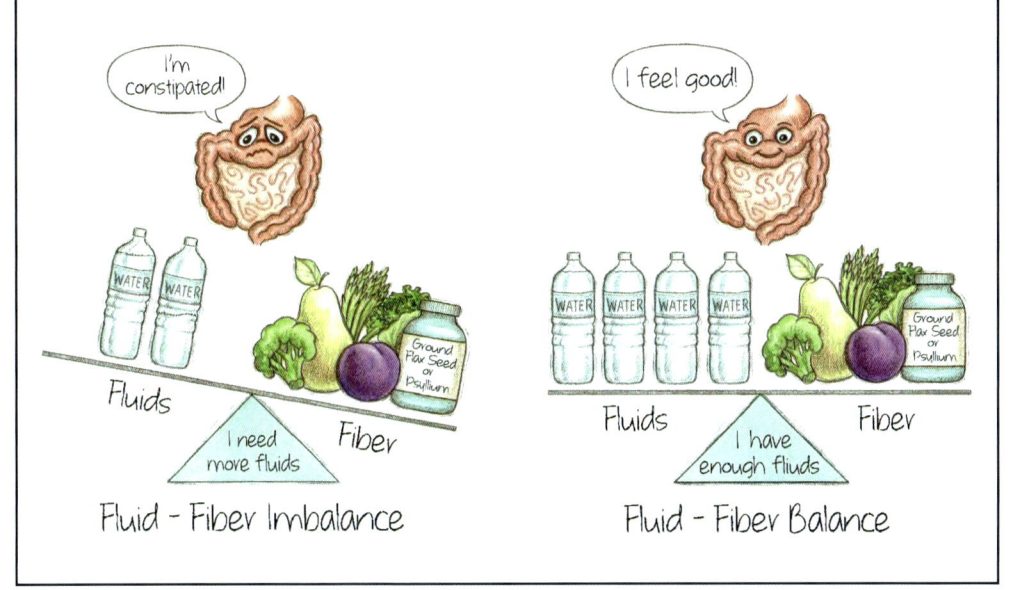

Fluid – Fiber Imbalance

Fluid – Fiber Balance

POOING WHILE TRAVELING

Why do I often get constipated while traveling?

A change in routine, sleep, and diet often causes a change in your poop (see my pellet poop story, page 49). When your routine is not regular, neither are your bowels. Try these poo tips while traveling:

Pre-load your pooing. The day before and the morning of travel, drink more *stoolade* (page 44).

Drink more water. Thirst is not always a reliable prompt to drink more fluids. Follow the fluid volume suggestions on page 43 and add an extra daily glass or two while traveling.

Take fiber along on your trip. See fiber supplement recommendations, page 57.

Move more. Sneak in at least 45 minutes of morning exercise and sneak in a few minutes of movement each hour during the day. Walk while you wait, such as before flight departures.

FODMAPs

I've heard that FODMAPs may be causing my tummy troubles. What are they and what do I need to know about reducing their consumption?

FODMAPs – an acronym for Fermentable Oligosaccharides, Disaccharides, Monosaccharides and Polyols – are simple, short-chain carbohydrates that may be poorly absorbed in the small intestine. Foods such as honey, pears, apples, watermelon, garlic, onions, cow's milk and lentils fall into this group. They are known to cause gas-related pain, bloating, constipation and/or diarrhea in people suffering from functional gastrointestinal disorders and irritable bowel syndrome. Reducing FODMAPs in the diet may reduce these symptoms.

Because many high-fiber foods are also high in FODMAPs, some people may have difficulty meeting their recommended daily fiber intake when following a low-FODMAP diet. This means they may not get enough soluble fiber which is essential for gut health and regularity. Many dietary fiber supplements, such as those made with inulin, wheat and corn dextrin, and IMOs are also high in FODMAPs, and should be avoided by those looking to reduce FODMAP consumption. Sunfiber and Regular Girl are two of the only commercially available fiber supplements that are Monash University Low FODMAP Certified™.

POO RULES – A SUMMARY

Holding hardens poop.

Go as soon as you feel the urge.

The sooner you go, the softer you poo.

The smaller your meals, the softer you poo.

A shake a day makes pooing ok.

The better you chew, the better you poo.

One to three poos a day keeps your gut feeling ok.

Poop should sink, not float.

Don't worry, just poo.

The less you poo, the more it smells.

Eating real good food makes real good poop.

Fiber-friendly food makes better poop.

Squat better, poo easier.

Dr. Poo's Chart

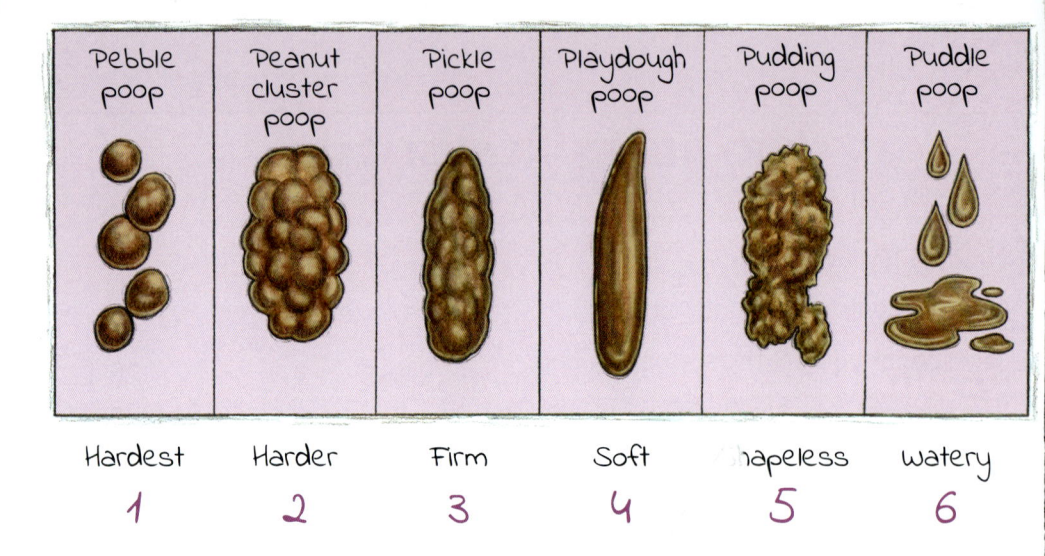

Pebble poop	Peanut cluster poop	Pickle poop	Playdough poop	Pudding poop	Puddle poop
Hardest	Harder	Firm	Soft	Shapeless	Watery
1	2	3	4	5	6

- Types one and two cause the most wear and tear on the rectal lining and require the most uncomfortable straining. Pebble poop can enlarge into golf-ball size or "plugged poop," which is the hardest to pass.

- Types three and four are usually the most comfortable poop. This soft poop is slippery and slides out naturally without much pushing, and tapers to a tail.

- Types five and six, if persistent, can signal that something is going on in your gut that needs medical attention. Or, it could be caused by some dietary intolerance or microbiome imbalance.

Your Poop is a Window into Your Health
Look before you flush!